Dementia-Friendly
Communities

of related interest

Living Well with Dementia through Music
A Resource Book for Activities Providers and Care Staff
Edited by Catherine Richards
Foreword by Helen Odell-Miller
ISBN 978 1 78592 488 0
eISBN 978 1 78450 878 4

Using Technology in Dementia Care
A Guide to Technology Solutions for Everyday Living
Edited by Professor Arlene Astell, Dr. Sarah Kate Smith and Dr. Phil Joddrell
ISBN 978 1 78592 417 0
eISBN 978 1 78450 779 4

Dementia – Support for Family and Friends, Second Edition
Dave Pulsford and Rachel Thompson
ISBN 978 1 78592 437 8
eISBN 978 1 78450 811 1

Sharing Sensory Stories and Conversations with People with Dementia
A Practical Guide
Joanna Grace
ISBN 978 1 78592 409 5
eISBN 978 1 78450 769 5

Essentials of Dementia
Everything You Really Need to Know for Working in Dementia Care
Dr. Shibley Rahman and Professor Rob Howard
Forewords by Karen Harrison Dening and by Kate Swaffer
ISBN 978 1 78592 397 5
eISBN 978 1 78450 754 1

Dementia-Friendly
Communities

Why We Need Them and
How We Can Create Them

Susan H. McFadden, PhD

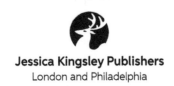

Jessica Kingsley Publishers
London and Philadelphia

First published in Great Britain in 2021 by Jessica Kingsley Publishers
An Hachette Company

1

Copyright © Susan H. McFadden, PhD 2021

The epigraph on p.47 is reproduced from Albee 2008 with kind permission from
William Morris Endeavor Entertainment, LLC. *The Zoo Story* Copyright © 1969 by
Edward Albee. *At Home at the Zoo* Copyright © 2008 by Edward Albee.

The epigraph on p.127 is reproduced from Rothe, Kruetzner & Gronemeyer 2017
with kind permission from Transcript Verlag.

The epigraph on p.169 is reproduced from Basting 2006 with kind permission from
the American Society on Aging.

Front cover image source: Shutterstock®.

A CIP catalogue record for this title is available from the British Library and the
Library of Congress

ISBN 978 1 78592 816 1
eISBN 978 1 78592 878 9

Printed and bound in the United States by Integrated Books International

Jessica Kingsley Publishers' policy is to use papers that are natural, renewable
and recyclable products and made from wood grown in sustainable forests. The
logging and manufacturing processes are expected to conform to the environmental
regulations of the country of origin.

Jessica Kingsley Publishers
Carmelite House
50 Victoria Embankment
London EC4Y 0DZ

www.jkp.com

Contents

Part 5: Embracing the New Story

Preface

Many of us have heard the stereotypes associated with people living with Alzheimer's disease or another dementia: that they are "no longer themselves," that they are "shells of their former selves." This common narrative focuses on degenerative processes in the brain coupled with the claim that dementia results not only in loss of selfhood but also in loss of humanity.

Of course, the suffering and losses experienced by persons living with dementia, by their families and friends, and by the people who interact with them in the wider community are very real. But I believe that there is another story to be told. This new narrative is about people working together in their communities to *disrupt* the assumptions about dementia that tell us that its symptoms are shameful and the condition hopeless.

I also believe that we need to disrupt the assumption that it is solely the responsibility of family members to offer care to people living with dementia. Today, most books about dementia focus on family "care partners," although some use the more widely recognized word "caregivers." This newer term, care partners, has gained wider use because it implies both that care requires a team (not a lone caregiver) and that the person living with dementia plays an active role in her own care. She not only participates in her care and decision-making as part of her care team, to the extent she is able, but also offers reciprocal care to those around her, which can be as simple as a smile or hug to show affection.

Such mutuality of caring can be expressed in many ways. For example, I once attended a community meeting called by several state legislators who were studying Wisconsin's dementia support systems. A couple I knew from our local memory café attended, and the wife, who cared for her husband with rather advanced dementia, signed in to speak to the legislators. I was sitting several rows back from the couple and observed that, when she was handed the microphone to speak from her seat, her husband reached over to rest his hand gently on her back. To me, that was an expression of a caring partnership.

Changes in family structures—such as divorce and remarriage, fewer children, and everyone's increased mobility—mean that care must be embedded in community programs and services acting in partnership with the care offered by family members and friends. That couple at the legislators' meeting had relocated to our community when he was diagnosed with Alzheimer's disease. They were some of the first people to attend our memory cafés. Even though they had an adult child living in our community, they reported that he was so busy with his work and family that they were not able to see him or his family as often as they had hoped. Quickly, however, through their participation in the memory café, they developed a network of friends who shared aspects of their dementia journey. This is not what they had expected when they moved to our community. Their expectations had been disrupted.

Until the dawn of the twenty-first century, disruption usually had a negative meaning related to the ways in which human lives are disrupted by broken relationships, diseases, poverty, natural disasters, and wars. Recently, however, a different, more positive light has illuminated the idea of disruption. The shift in thinking about disruption arose in descriptions of new technologies and businesses disrupting everything from how we communicate to how we clean our homes.[1] Those new technologies and businesses put telephones in our pockets that have more functions than we could have imagined when we got our first bulky desktop computers, and some people now have little robots that scoot all over their floors and eliminate the task of pushing heavy vacuum cleaners.

Reflecting this more positive view of disruption, some people have begun talking about disrupting dementia with a new vision that calls for partnering with people living with dementia[2] in order to provide the kind of good life they want in their communities. These partnerships represent the foundation for dementia inclusiveness.

This means that community programs and services for people living with dementia will be based on the expressed needs and desires of the people they are designed to serve.

The notion of disruption through technology and through changes in typical responses to dementia converged in 2016 at the enormous Consumer Electronics Show held annually in Las Vegas, Nevada. Technology entrepreneurs had the opportunity to attend sessions billed as presenting ways of disrupting dementia through technological innovations. A year later, Dr. Bill Thomas, founder of The Eden Alternative and The Green House Project (which intended to radically reform the culture of long-term care), created the Age of Disruption Tour, which includes a workshop called "Disrupt Dementia." It features music and storytelling by people living with dementia.[3]

The diagnosis of dementia, or even the suspicion of dementia, can dramatically disrupt people's lives in a negative way. New technologies can also have a negative impact on everyday life, such as the feeling of being unable to escape from the 24/7 stream of messages coming through smartphones. Although the notion of disrupting dementia is intended to be a positive turn away from the gloom and doom of much dementia discourse, as well as a rejection of inhumane forms of care, there is still something unsettling about disruption. We must hold two ideas in creative tension: that dementia causes considerable disturbing disruption, and that people can retain a sense of dignity and hold on to hope when their communities offer opportunities for forming and sustaining meaningful relationships.

In the 1980s, when I became a professor of psychology, I tried to help my students understand the interwoven dynamics of loss and gain in later life. They had no trouble articulating what they viewed as the losses of aging, but they had trouble naming anything that might be gained. They began to understand how people could experience both when I asked them to think about losses and gains in childhood and adolescence. Then, they easily produced examples such as losing the sweet comfort of cuddling on a parent's lap but gaining enough independence to ride a bicycle without a parent nearby. Eventually, they understood that an older person might lose physical agility but gain patience and compassion. These students also began to see that some loss is good and some gain is bad, and that human life is a complex, often mysterious, mixture of loss and gain, good and bad. Very often, however, people find that mixture—that gray zone—too uncomfortable and resort to splitting loss and gain, or good and bad, into opposing camps.

In the 1990s, I noticed a lot of splitting occurring in gerontology. At conferences, presentations on aspects of so-called "successful aging" would be separated in the program from presentations on aging with chronic conditions such as dementia. The idea of successful aging took hold after the publication of a book by John W. Rowe and Robert L. Kahn. They claimed that to age successfully, one needed to have low risk of disease and disability, high cognitive and physical abilities, and meaningful engagement with others.[4] I wondered whether that meant that having dementia implied a person had failed at aging. Was it possible for someone to meet the criteria for successful aging and also have some form of dementia? Now that we are 20 years into the twenty-first century, I am still navigating through the gray zone between acknowledging the suffering and loss and continuing to remain hopeful that life can still be good despite a dementia diagnosis. As illustrated by the quotes I include later from people living with the diagnosis, this hope depends upon meaningful relationships with others that affirm their dignity.

Overview of the Book

In Part 1 of this book, I present an introduction to the new story that can disrupt the common view of dementia. When I describe my work with people living with dementia, I frequently encounter people who say, "Oh, that's so depressing" and "There's no cure, so what can we do?" and "I sure hope I never have dementia." Chapter 1 describes the demographics and attitudes that often lead to statements such as these. Chapter 2 offers a brief introduction to dementia and answers the frequently asked question "What is the difference between Alzheimer's and dementia?" Chapter 3 rounds out the introduction by offering a brief history of how we moved from assuming that senility is a typical outcome of growing old—an assumption that originated in a time when few people actually did grow old—to the currently emerging view that dementia does not rob people of their rights as citizens to participate in their communities.

Part 2 begins where all discussions of dementia policies, programs, and services should start: with persons living with this condition. Chapter 4 introduces people who are living as well as possible with this frustrating, stigmatized, and terminal condition. Themes from their work reveal the ways they articulate hope—especially hope for how they can continue to be treated with dignity and be included in their communities. Chapter 5 describes how they advocate for the preservation of dignity and human rights for all persons living with dementia through their dementia activism.

Part 3 offers ideas about friendship and inclusion, showing in Chapter 6 how friends can help to disrupt dementia once they realize that it is possible to remain in friendship with someone who may no longer recall the story of the friendship. Chapter 7 moves from the closeness of friendship to the wider community and addresses various ways of defining and experiencing community. Chapter 8 reviews practical issues raised by the desire to create dementia-inclusive and friendly communities; it is the "how-to" chapter.

In Part 4, I attempt to broaden the discussion by addressing two topics of critical importance to any discussion of living well with dementia: the arts and spirituality. Chapter 9 describes collaborations with artists who are bringing engagement with various art forms into all types of dementia care. Chapter 10 offers a model of spirituality that includes the arts as well as more traditional expressions of religiousness, and it shows how faith communities can play an important role in encouraging communities to disrupt dementia through practices of inclusivity.

In Part 5, I conclude this new story about dementia by returning to the themes of hope and dignity. Just one chapter, Part 5 reviews key points from previous chapters and suggests new directions for dementia research, practice, and policy. They help us address key questions about hope and dignity, such as

- For what can we hope?

- How can those who love persons with dementia hold on to hope in the face of so much loss and suffering?

- What do people living with dementia hope for, both for themselves and for their communities?

That last question invites us to consider what dignity means and how friends and communities can uphold the dignity and human rights of all persons regardless of their cognitive capacity.

Endnotes

1   One of the first widely available works on disruption in the business world is a book that can be downloaded for free. This, in itself, is disruptive.

   Christensen, C. M. (1997). *The innovator's dilemma: When new technologies cause great firms to fail*. Boston, MA: Harvard Business School Press.

2   Throughout the book, when I talk about people "living with dementia," I am referring to diagnosed persons, care partners, friends, and others whose lives are affected by dementia. In truth, I am referring to most of us.

3   The tour was inspired by AARP's goal of disrupting aging and by the work of Momentia, an organization in Seattle working to improve the quality of life for people living with dementia. Descriptions of the tour and brief videos can be found at https://changingaging.org/tour/disrupt-dementia

4   Rowe and Kahn's book set off a storm of controversy in gerontology. It became well known quickly, probably due in part to the fact that the MacArthur Foundation, which funded the research, sent free copies to many academic gerontologists.

   Rowe, J. W., & Kahn, R. L. (1998). *Successful aging*. New York, NY: Pantheon Books.

Part 1

TELLING A NEW STORY

Chapter 1

The Current Situation

Diagnosed at age 50, Peter Berry is now several years into his new life with younger-onset Alzheimer's disease, which affects people age 65 and under. After the diagnosis, when he hit his lowest point, he concluded, "The world would be a better place without me." Since then, Peter has met many people who experience that feeling upon receiving this dreaded diagnosis.

Fortunately, Peter experienced a dramatic attitude shift when he realized he could help others live a decent life by sharing his experiences. This insight pulled him out of that low place. In one of his weekly YouTube videos about living with dementia, he states, "It is a terrible disease, but if you can live life in a positive way and if you can achieve things, you might be able to live longer and better."

In the summer of 2018, Peter rode his bicycle 330 miles across England to raise money for YoungDementia UK. He says that cycling enables him to "leave dementia at home for a while." He acknowledges his dark days, but he also describes how he returns to the "power of being positive" and the effects that attitude can have on others.[1]

On YouTube, in posts on Twitter accounts such as @YoungDementiaUK and Facebook groups like MemoryPeople, as well as in blogs and books, people with dementia are speaking out about how they cope with a diagnosis that is feared more than cancer. They know that they have a progressive condition that affects memory and other cognitive abilities, but they also know that they still experience a wide range of emotions. They are advocating for themselves, offering support to strangers living with similar diagnoses, and insisting that their local communities support dementia-inclusive initiatives. Even those who do not regularly access social media are engaging in forms of dementia-inclusive community advocacy by urging local businesses and organizations to train employees, through programs such as the Purple Angel Dementia Awareness Campaign, to offer compassionate, patient service to persons living with dementia.[2]

Peter Berry and others living with some type of dementia are determined not to disappear from their communities. They insist on being given the opportunity to live as well as possible with a condition that challenges the assumptions of what ethicist Stephen Post calls our "hypercognitive culture."[3] They want their communities to be

- *aware* of how to remain in relationship with people having dementia

- *friendly* toward diagnosed persons and their care partners

- *capable* of providing supportive environments and trained staff (particularly in health-care settings)

- *positive* about possibilities for living well with dementia

- and thus *enabling* individuals to enjoy life by providing *inclusive* community resources.[4]

These courageous, outspoken individuals will not fade away quietly. And yet, despite the emerging activism by people like Peter Berry, much of the general public still expects those with dementia to passively accept being locked away and out of sight. This is why Berry and others introduced in this book are disrupting dementia by telling a new story about dementia. They want to remain included in community life regardless of their dementia diagnosis. They know the great disruption that a dementia diagnosis injects into people's lives, but they also know that personal disruption can be cushioned when family members, friends, and people in their communities embrace the new story and disrupt prevalent social attitudes about dementia.

The new narrative of dementia is being told in many communities, although the old narrative remains dominant. The new story includes a broad range of images of dementia, from Peter on his bicycle to Marie who lives at The Elms, a memory-care residence.[5]

The Elms is a specialized, secure (locked) assisted-living community with activities designed for people living with dementia and staff trained in dementia care. Marie has lived there for two years. She cannot create her own YouTube channel, but she can still hold her husband's hand, smile when greeted, and tap her foot as she listens to a chorus of people whose dementia has not progressed as much as hers. Marie's language is limited, but she is still able to communicate that she feels blessed by the love and care she receives at The Elms.

The old dementia story offers a dismal portrayal of Marie and those like her, a story that many people would rather not hear and that often gets generalized to people like Peter who have not relocated to some type of care community. Those who have not crossed the threshold of a nursing home since childhood when they visited Grandma may still conjure images of unkempt old people slouched in wheelchairs with *Wheel of Fortune* blaring in the background. Sadly, this image is still an accurate portrayal of some places. However, the culture-change movement inspired in the late 1990s by Tom Kitwood, a British psychologist, has positively affected the programs, architecture, and mission of many long-term care organizations.

Learning about Kitwood's work was a life-changing event for me. I had been doing research at a continuing-care retirement community (CCRC) near my university. My students and I were studying residents' responses to a move from a section of the CCRC built in the 1960s with long, narrow hallways, double rooms, and a central nursing station. The new part of the CCRC featured four households, each having 11 residents with private rooms and their own bathrooms. All residents had some type of dementia. Each household had a central living area integrated with a kitchen and dining area. Today, many care communities employ this design, but in the late 1990s it was considered innovative. The CCRC's executive director had led the push for the new addition, and he encouraged researchers to investigate its effects on residents. In the summer of 1998, the executive director invited about 40 people to come from all over the United States to Oshkosh, Wisconsin, to continue the work they had begun the previous year to create the Pioneer Network™.[6] The Network's goal is to change the culture of aging, particularly for elders living in some type of long-term care residence.

Our meeting in 1998 had a positive disruptive vibe. For example, unlike at most conferences, no one wore a nametag with academic degrees. Thus, you could not know if you were talking with a physician, a certified nursing assistant, a social worker, or the owner of a nursing home. Also, we participated in rituals involving music and movement designed to help us connect with one another and focus on the opportunities and challenges of transforming long-term care. I was not used to singing and dancing at professional meetings.

Kitwood's book *Dementia Reconsidered*[7] described person-centered care. His subtitle, "the person comes first," reflected his insistence that the person with dementia be heard and respected. He contrasted person-centered care with the old-culture idea that only medical professionals really understand or can speak for the person with dementia. Old-culture care was just about meeting basic needs. The new culture of care honors the personhood of residents. Inspired by the work of the Jewish philosopher and theologian Martin Buber, Kitwood argued that personhood is born in relationships. Without recognition of personhood, people tend to regard an individual with dementia as an "It" (capitalized by Buber) and to treat that person an object, rather than as a "Thou" to be appreciated as fully human. In addition to urging a new perspective about long-term care residents, Kitwood also said that the people actually doing the caring—the nursing assistants and other poorly paid employees— have important knowledge grounded in experience. Their voices need to be heard. Kitwood emphasized that care is about enhancing personhood through meaningful relationships, and that having these relationships is just as much a basic need as food and safety.

Returning to Marie's story, Marie's long-term-care community supports meaningful relationships with family members, staff, and community volunteers. It encourages staff to take time to get to know residents, provides frequent opportunities for enjoyable interactions through creative-engagement programs, and regularly offers activities such as picnics, concerts, and lectures that welcome community members. In addition, residents like Marie often ride through town on a cargo bike called a trishaw that has seats in the back for two and is pedaled by a trained volunteer.[8] Marie and her friends can wave to children playing in parks, neighbors chatting, people washing their cars, and folks drinking coffee outdoors at cafés. Some of these people volunteer regularly at The Elms by leading singing groups, guiding art projects, and helping residents create stories and poems.

Human beings are storytellers. We create narratives that set individual lives within broader cultural themes. Those themes sometimes seem to be set in stone—but they are not. They can be changed because human storytellers have the capacity to shift their narratives.

Communities need to hear this new story for the sake of all whose lives are touched by dementia. And the demographics of dementia suggest that the "all" in my last sentence refers to nearly everyone.

Big Numbers

According to the US Census Bureau, 2020 marks the year of a worldwide crossover event with the number of people 65 and older exceeding the number of children less than five years old.[9] This is unprecedented in human history. Because age is the greatest risk factor for dementia, not only will there be many more older people but also there will be more people living with Alzheimer's disease and other types of dementia.

By 2050, the world population of persons 65 and older will be twice the number of children younger than five. With no cure in sight for the many types of dementia, this means that more people will find themselves living with symptoms that can include recall dysfunction (usually called memory loss), problems with decision-making, difficulties managing everyday life activities, and, in some cases, personality change. This phenomenon will be felt most acutely in Asia, Europe, Oceania, and the US.[10]

In the US, the Alzheimer's Association estimates that about 5.8 million Americans currently live with some form of dementia, the most common being Alzheimer's dementia.[11] Differentiation of the more familiar term "Alzheimer's disease" from the newer term "Alzheimer's dementia" resulted from a report in 2011 by a workgroup organized by the US National Institute on Aging and the Alzheimer's Association (NIA/AA).[12] The NIA/AA group recommended separate diagnostic descriptions of three stages of Alzheimer's disease: preclinical (no symptoms, but identifiable brain changes), mild cognitive impairment (some noticeable symptoms that do not interfere with ordinary life), and dementia (symptoms accompanied by changes in daily functioning due to specific problems with cognition, emotion, and motivation).

The term "Alzheimer's disease" is used in two ways. To refer to the third stage when symptoms interfere with everyday life as "Alzheimer's disease" is the most common. However, under the new guidelines, "Alzheimer's disease" can apply to persons whose brains may have the kind of pathology first identified by Dr. Alois Alzheimer in 1906, but they do not have the typical symptoms of dementia (and, in fact, they may never develop the symptoms). According to this approach, one might have "Alzheimer's disease" long before one has "Alzheimer's dementia." For this reason, some researchers now say we should think of Alzheimer's disease as a disease of midlife, not old age. I occasionally shock college students and community groups when I give talks and declare, "I may have Alzheimer's disease."

Although the number of people living in the US with Alzheimer's dementia is widely publicized, it obscures several important factors. First, no one really knows how many people actually have Alzheimer's and other types of dementia, because only about half of all people with dementia symptoms receive a diagnosis based on careful medical and neuropsychological testing. Second, less than half of Medicare beneficiaries who have a diagnosis in their medical record are ever informed about it. Finally, current studies report that about 4 percent of adults younger than 65 may have some form of dementia, but because so few of them receive a diagnosis, this number is uncertain. In short, Alzheimer's and other dementias are under-diagnosed and underreported; and with a growing population of people living past 65, the number of people living with dementia will increase dramatically by 2050.[13] By that year, it is estimated that in the US, 51 percent of people age 85 and older will have Alzheimer's dementia. This does not include individuals with other types of dementia.[14]

We need to consider the implications of these big numbers for local communities and their citizens who live with dementia. In the US, almost half of all persons with some form of dementia receive care from a family member or friend, although that number is considerably higher among some culturally and linguistically diverse groups in the US, and in many other countries. This unpaid care has been estimated at a value of over \$230 billion for the US economy.[15] These care partners often have either to leave the workforce or to reduce their hours in order to provide care, thus affecting their own economic security.

Sometimes, despite the courageous efforts of care partners to meet all the needs of a person living with dementia, symptoms may become unmanageable. Washing bedding several times a day, responding to calls for help all through the night, fears about a loved one wandering from home, struggles over bathing and other personal hygiene, concerns about nutrition, and sheer exhaustion— stressors such as these can force care partners to turn to some form of paid home care or residential care, if they can afford it. And yet it is hard to imagine, given the demographic projections for the next few decades, that there will be enough good-quality care facilities to meet the growing need. Nor will many families in the US be able to pay the bills, because Medicare, which is designed to pay for acute-care needs, does not cover most long-term home or residential care.[16]

An even thornier question concerns whether building more care communities for individuals with dementia is the best approach. Can we really imagine a world in which millions of persons with dementia move out of their homes and into some type of residential care? After all, one of the hallmarks of any form of dementia is that it is a progressive, terminal condition. Thus, as symptoms become more challenging, more assistance will be needed. However, even if it were possible to build and fund a sufficient number of care facilities where people with dementia could live through the last stages of life, would that be the best solution for those persons, their families, and their communities?

Beyond the consideration of physical buildings and paying for care, there is another important issue. Who will work in these places, especially given the fact that the proportion of younger persons in many countries is dropping compared with people 65 and older? Not only will there be fewer individuals to work in various types of residential care settings (a problem currently felt acutely in many parts of the world, including the US), but it will be increasingly difficult to attract younger people to do this work because the pay is so low.

These numbers are real—and they can elicit a sense of dread about a future with so many older individuals with dementia. Sometimes, experts talk about how this condition will "bankrupt" society and produce a terrible "burden" that all will have to bear. In other words, the personhood of individuals having dementia, and the love and care most families offer, is swept aside and replaced with arguments about who will pay the bills and with living arrangements that remove affected persons from their communities.

This bleak narrative is dangerous because it can quickly lead some to conclude that societies would be better off if there were no people living with dementia. This "put them on an iceberg" fantasy must be directly addressed, analyzed, and repudiated. Although dementia is too often presented as a hopeless condition that robs people of their dignity, many have found that hope and dignity can flourish when communities intentionally affirm and support the human rights and humanity of all persons.

A Case for Social Change

In order that people might tell and experience this new story of hope and dignity for people living with dementia, significant social changes must occur on several levels of public life. On an individual level, we must change the way we talk about dementia. This will not be easy, for the habit of casting dementia only in the language of dread and despair is strongly ingrained. However, changing language alongside structural social change can have a powerful effect on attitudes. For example, in the early twentieth century, medical practitioners categorized some children as morons, imbeciles, or idiots depending on their scores on intelligence tests. Later, as that language faded, the term "mental retardation" was widely adopted, until it, too, became pejorative, with people being called "retards." Although stigma about developmental disability[17] remains, schools and social-service organizations work hard to emphasize the strengths of persons living with various genetic or physical causes contributing to low scores on intelligence tests.

The change in language about persons with developmental

disabilities coincided with changes in attitudes and social policies. Until late in the twentieth century, physicians advised parents of children born with obvious signs of intellectual disability to place them in state-run institutions, a practice we reject today, as schools and workplaces have adapted to serve these individuals. When parents became politically active as advocates for their children's needs for education and meaningful work, institutional and policy changes followed.

The attitudinal, institutional, and policy changes that now support persons with intellectual disabilities who live, love, learn, and work in our communities may come more slowly to those advocating for similar social change for people living with mental-health problems and with dementia. Although adults need not concern themselves with becoming developmentally disabled, as such conditions arise in childhood, many of us still worry that we may be diagnosed with depression or debilitating anxiety. Social exclusion of people with mental-health problems occurs in part because of fears about associating with individuals whose life circumstances remind us that we, too, could succumb to mental illness. Even more frightening is the fact that getting older brings a higher risk of developing some type of dementia.

Such fears about dementia have many sources. Descartes' conviction that his thinking proved his being ("I think, therefore I am") influenced Western culture's emphasis on cognitive capacity as a reflection of personal worth and value. Confusion in thinking, inability to remember newly acquired information, impaired decision-making, and other indications of problems with cognition—in particular, difficulties with executive function— have been interpreted as proof that a person's selfhood has been diminished. One 2011 publication about the threat of dementia for the baby-boom generation even stated that in its final stages "Alzheimer's robs people of all bodily functions and eventually their humanity."[18]

Leaders of the culture-change movement understand that dehumanizing statements such as that one have had profound negative consequences for people with dementia living in residential care homes. They assert that culture change within these residences has to involve more than architectural alterations to make them appear more homelike and less like medical institutions. They advocate for interpersonal relationships that honor and support the personhood of each resident. They also insist on honoring and supporting the personhood of the often poorly paid employees who provide the most direct care. Unfortunately, for a long time these ideas did not always gain traction, either within the large organizations that purchased many formerly independent care homes (organizations that argued that economies of scale would help to address the high costs of care within "the industry") or with the public that retained frightening images of nursing homes.

Slowly but surely, however, ideas about culture change and personhood are spreading through long-term care organizations as well as public discourse about good life quality for people living with dementia regardless of where they reside. In other words, although culture change initially focused on the culture of care residences, we now see a broader understanding taking hold as efforts to create dementia-friendly communities proliferate.

One major challenge for the future will be to demonstrate how a social model of dementia can help us understand the ways "attitudes, environments and policies make life harder for people with dementia (and their families)."[19] It will be insufficient for a community simply to call itself "dementia-friendly." The hard work of identifying and eliminating social barriers will need to be undertaken, along with critical examination of the denial of certain human rights for people with dementia.

As noted at the beginning of this chapter, this social change is driven in part by persons living with the diagnosis, as they continue to speak up about what they need from community partners. It is also driven by educators teaching and doing research on aging, old age, and older adults; by artists discovering exciting opportunities to share creative-expression activities with people living with dementia; by clergy realizing how many of their congregants are living with dementia; by social workers seeing how dementia affects multiple generations in families; and by politicians hearing from constituents about the need for policies, supported by budgets, that enable people to live as well as possible despite their diagnosis.

All of these social changes are disrupting the narrative that people with dementia experience a loss of self and even humanity. But unlike with some other recent social and technological disruptions, I see no negative consequences of eliminating dementia stigma, creating inclusive communities, and supporting the kinds of programs that enable people with dementia, care partners, and paid caregivers to live as good a life as possible (unless, of course, one were to consider it a negative consequence to have to pay for these programs). All of us can disrupt dementia by accepting it as a disability that can be accommodated in a variety of ways that not only benefit people with the disability but also benefit the wider society. After all, who would not want to live in a community that offers opportunities for hope and dignity to be experienced by all citizens?

Endnotes

1   Peter Berry introduces himself, the story of being diagnosed with younger-onset Alzheimer's dementia, and his bike riding in this YouTube video: www.youtube.com/watch?v=cVjxooR3_2M

2   The Purple Angel Dementia Awareness Campaign resulted when Norman McNamara was diagnosed with Lewy body dementia. He decided he needed to resist the stigma of his diagnosis by training businesses and other organizations in his community (Devon, UK) to offer better service to people with dementia. He soon began collaborating with Jane Moore, a woman in Cornwall, UK, caring for her "mum" with dementia. The Purple Angel campaign has now spread internationally. For more information, see www.purpleangel-global.com

3   Stephen Post's book challenges common assumptions about personhood rooted in Descartes' assertion that "I think, therefore I am." What happens to personhood when an individual can no longer demonstrate rational thinking, memory for recent events, problem-solving, etc.? Those seeking to transform communities to be dementia inclusive must engage deeply with this question.

      Post, S. (2000). *The moral challenge of Alzheimer disease: Ethical issues from diagnosis to dying* (2nd ed.). Baltimore, MD: Johns Hopkins University Press.

4   All of these italicized words appear in articles and books describing new thinking about how people can live as well as possible with dementia.

5   All references in this book to people I know use pseudonyms. The names of the places where they live have been changed.

6   The original name was Pioneers in Nursing Home Culture Change. About 35 people from eight states and DC met in Rochester, NY, in March 1997. Bill Thomas attended and led a ritual to acknowledge Carter Catlett Williams as the original convener of the Pioneer Movement. The following year, at the 1998 meeting, attendees presented a quilt to Carter consisting of pieces each person contributed. This is the origin of the quilt logo for Pioneer Network: www.pioneernetwork.net

7   Kitwood, T. (1997). *Dementia reconsidered: The person comes first*. Philadelphia, PA: Open University Press.

8   Begun in 2012 in Copenhagen, Denmark, the Cycling Without Age program has spread throughout the world to enable elders, including those living with dementia, to "feel the wind in their hair" and remain connected to their communities. See: https://cyclingwithoutage.org

9   He, W., Goodkind, D., & Kowal, P. (2016). *An aging world: 2015.* Washington, DC: US Government Publishing Office. Accessed on 7/12/19 at www.census.gov/content/dam/Census/library/publications/2016/demo/p95-16-1.pdf

10 He et al.

11 The Alzheimer's Association publishes annual reports on prevalence and incidence of dementia as well as related topics such as caregiving, health care, long-term care, morbidity, and mortality.
    Alzheimer's Association. (2019). Alzheimer's disease facts and figures. *Alzheimer's & Dementia, 15*(3), 321–387. Accessed on 9/26/19 at www.alz.org/media/documents/alzheimers-facts-and-figures-2019-r.pdf

12 Jack, C. R. Jr., Albert, M. S., Knopman, D. S., McKhann, G. M., Sperling, R. A., Carillo, M., et al. (2011). Introduction to the recommendations from the National Institute on Aging–Alzheimer's Association workgroups on diagnostic guidelines for Alzheimer's disease. *Alzheimer's & Dementia, 7,* 257–262.

13 Alzheimer's Association (2019).

14 Hebert, L. E., Weuve, J., Scherr, P. A., & Evans, D. A. (2013). Alzheimer disease in the United States (2010–2050) estimated using the 2010 census. *Neurology, 80,* 1778–1783.

15 Alzheimer's Association (2019).

16 Here is a personal example. I am blessed by friendship with a 98-year-old woman who, while not living with dementia, has multiple health challenges. She has been homebound in an apartment for four years due to a persistent wound on her foot that required a weekly trip to a wound nurse and her own wound care on two other days of the week. She was getting along with Meals on Wheels and a home-care aide who came for two hours, twice a week, to do light chores, pick up prescriptions, etc. When my friend fell and broke her dominant arm by her shoulder socket, she could no longer use her walker, button her shirt, or do other self-care tasks. She was told to get 24/7 care in her apartment, but when she discovered that would cost $18,000 a month, she realized she needed another approach. Fortunately, I was able to help her get admitted to an assisted-living residence where she paid about $4,800 a month in addition to the rent for her apartment to which she eventually returned.

17 Many types of chronic conditions contribute to developmental disabilities that affect physical and/or mental functioning and are obvious before adulthood. Sometimes, people use the term "intellectual disabilities," and, currently, it is common to see references to "I/DD" in order to include both developmental and intellectual disabilities. Down syndrome is one of the best-known examples. Because more people with I/DD are living longer, some—especially those with Down syndrome—develop Alzheimer's disease. In Massachusetts, Jewish Family & Children's Service has developed memory cafés specifically designed for these individuals. See this YouTube video for more information: www.youtube.com/watch?v=EE49z4CpyP8. Also, the National Task Group on Intellectual Disabilities and Dementia Practices has produced an excellent, comprehensive report that describes the persons and their challenges, as well as new thinking about community services for them: National Task Group on Intellectual Disabilities and Dementia Practices (2012). *"My Thinker's Not Working": A national strategy for enabling adults with intellectual disabilities affected by dementia to remain in their community and receive quality*

supports. Accessed on 7/2/20 at www.nursinghometoolkit.com/additionalresources/ MyThinkersNotWorking.pdf

18 Alzheimer's Association. (2011). *Generation Alzheimer's: The defining disease of the baby boomers.* Chicago, IL: Alzheimer's Association, p. 4. Accessed on 7/16/19 at http://act.alz.org/site/DocServer/ALZ_BoomersReport.pdf?docID=521

19 Shakespeare, T., Zeilig, H., & Mittler, P. (2019). Rights in mind: Thinking differently about dementia and disability. *Dementia, 18,* 1075–1088. (p. 1080)

Chapter 2

A Brief Introduction
to Dementia

In 2013, my husband, John, and I gave a talk on the importance of friendship and community connections for living well with dementia. We had been asked to present on this topic at the annual Meeting of the Minds conference sponsored by the Alzheimer's Association of Minnesota and North Dakota and by Mayo Clinic.

The day began with several sessions attended by everyone registered for the conference—over one thousand people. I vividly recall being in a large conference-center auditorium with huge screens, flashing purple lights (the color of Alzheimer's Association branding), and loud sound. I wondered how the people in the audience who were living with mild cognitive impairment (MCI) or the early stages of Alzheimer's disease or other types of dementia felt about an event that resembled a rock-and-roll concert. Many probably loved it, but others may have found it overwhelming.

The first plenary session of the day opened with an Alzheimer's Association video highlighting projections of the number of persons who will be diagnosed with Alzheimer's in the coming years. Then, with assistance from a former player on one of her storied teams, Pat Summitt, the renowned University of Tennessee basketball coach, spoke about her diagnosis of younger-onset Alzheimer's disease. Other speakers included Dr. Ronald Petersen of Mayo Clinic, who spoke about his pioneering research on MCI.

In our own presentation in a breakout session later that day, we included a PowerPoint slide that listed different types of dementia, of which there are over 100. I thought of this slide as merely informative, not as something that could create a lasting memory that sits alongside my recollection of the purple lights and booming sounds. But after our presentation, several people engaged us in conversations about what we had discussed. I noticed a couple standing quietly to the side of the room, waiting to approach us and looking at an iPad. I was surprised when they showed us that they were looking at the slide about dementia types. I was even more surprised when the husband began by saying, "Thank you." They told us that their initial impression of the conference, as they had sat through the welcoming remarks and the earlier speakers, was that they might not be welcome. They had asked themselves, "Are we different from the other people here? Should we leave?"

In our brief conversation, we learned that this couple were dealing with the wife's primary progressive aphasia (PPA), a form of frontotemporal dementia that in the early stages affects the ability to communicate. They wanted us to know that our single slide showing that there are many types of dementia made them feel as if their day would not be wasted.

The "Alzheimerization of Dementia"

This was my first experience of people feeling excluded because of what Dr. Bruce Miller, a leading researcher on frontotemporal dementia, calls the "Alzheimerization of dementia."[1] That couple, and many others like them, have taught me the importance of acknowledging individual differences not only in the type of dementia a person might have but also in the ways symptoms are expressed, the awareness the person has of the symptoms, and that person's relationships with others. The fact that every human being is a unique individual often gets ignored when the dementia label is acquired.

The year before I attended this conference in Minnesota, I noticed something odd in the National Plan to Address Alzheimer's Disease. It was published by the US Department of Health and Human Services and approved by Congress in 2012 in support of the National Alzheimer's Project Act (NAPA) signed by President Obama in 2011. The first goal of NAPA was to "create and maintain an integrated National Plan to overcome Alzheimer's disease." The other bullet points outlining the goals also referred to Alzheimer's disease. However, on page 4 of the plan, this statement appeared:

> In this plan, the term "Alzheimer's disease," or AD, refers to Alzheimer's disease and related dementias, consistent with the approach Congress used in NAPA. Related dementias include frontotemporal, Lewy body, mixed, and vascular dementia. It is often difficult to distinguish between Alzheimer's disease and other dementias in terms of clinical presentation and diagnosis. Some of the basic neurodegenerative processes have common pathways. People with dementia and their families face similar challenges in finding appropriate and necessary medical and supportive care. Unless otherwise noted, in this plan AD refers to these conditions collectively.[2]

This inclusion of all forms of dementia in the category "Alzheimer's disease" is an example of what drove that couple at the Minnesota conference to feel excluded.

A slight shift in the terminology of the National Plan to Address Alzheimer's Disease has occurred since its first appearance in 2012. In the update released in 2018, one now finds acknowledgment of other forms of dementia through the use of the term "Alzheimer's Disease and Related Dementias" (ADRD). However, the updated National Plan states the goal of overcoming "AD/ADRD"[3] and refers to AD/ADRD throughout the document. In other words, Alzheimer's disease got double billing!

Contrast this with England's national dementia plan that appeared in 2009. It was titled *Living Well with Dementia* and stated that its vision was to "improve the quality of life for people with dementia and their carers."[4] The vision for the US plan, on the other hand, was to "eliminate the burden of Alzheimer's disease." Presumably, eliminating burden can improve quality of life, but emphasizing burden immediately shifts the narrative toward the negative.

It cannot be denied that dementia burdens people with the diagnosis and their care partners, and it is hard to imagine a time when government policies and programs would free people entirely from burden. Anyone in any important relationship (spouse, partner, parent, friend, coworker, etc.) knows that meaningful connections with others sometimes produce burdens. This is part of the human condition. Certainly burdens can be eased, and often that happens when people agree to share burdens. For example, a friend might offer to take a husband with dementia to a memory café so his wife can enjoy an afternoon of self-care. These kinds of individual actions contribute to an improved quality of life, and on a wider scale, dementia-inclusive communities enable and support this kind of burden sharing.

Returning to the two national plans, although there are some similarities, one glaring difference can be seen immediately on their covers. The US plan has a plain blue cover with its official title printed in a white space. The English plan features color photographs of several people with dementia. Its cover also includes this phrase: "Putting People First." Another big difference is the language used in the plans. While the US plan revision from 2018 talks about AD/ADRD, the English plan refers to "the dementias."

"The Dementias" and "A Dementia"

What a difference small, common words and a single letter can make. In some writing, mostly by people working in the humanities, reference to "the dementias" is starting to catch on, because this recognizes that there are many types of dementia. Similarly, I occasionally see articles about people living with *a* dementia.[5] As I will note throughout this book, the language we use to talk about the dementias exerts a powerful influence. It affects how people think, and the feelings they have, about the condition and the people who live with it.

For example, some people believe that when we describe individual persons living with dementia as living with "a dementia" we are beginning to move dementia into the category of disability. Just as we are now quite used to referring to a disabled person as having "a disability" specific to them, some argue that using "a" before "dementia" gives a person a similar dignity by clarifying that different types of dementias present different challenges and day-to-day realities. No one wants to be lumped into a broad category, as that is another way to feel invisible.

But such linkage of the term "a dementia" with disability is new and controversial. Many people would resist the label "disabled" just as strongly as they object to being called demented. Moreover, the disability rights community has not yet embraced the idea that people with a type of dementia should join their movement. A recent paper, however, illustrates how this attitude may be shifting. The three authors describe themselves as a person living with a disability, a person living with a mental-health condition, and a person living with dementia. They assert that inviting people with dementia into the world of disability activism "means reconfiguring our approaches to disability as a whole."[6] For example, typical views of disability assume that both the disability and the feelings and needs of the person living with the disability are fairly static. This perspective does not take aging into account and the fact that people living with dementia have emotions and needs that change over time, something that is true for all human beings regardless of their mental or physical condition. These authors note that calling dementia a disability might also benefit the disability community by challenging that community

> to remember how impairments can impact daily living, and how emotionality is important. It also reminds us how humans can communicate and connect without language, and that we are more than our memories.[7]

Beyond the complex, controversial issues of what constitutes a disability and who should be included in efforts to secure social acceptance for people with disabilities, the general public seems to have come to accept—and often to appreciate—the accommodations that make it possible for persons with a disability to live as well as possible. The curb cuts that enable people using wheelchairs to get around their neighborhoods benefit people pushing strollers. The automated voices activated by pressing buttons at crosswalks benefit blind persons and remind everyone that it is safe to proceed. In a similar way, efforts to create dementia-friendly and inclusive communities gain strength when we recognize that physical and social accommodations that make a big difference for people living with dementia "will be felt not just by those living with dementia, but by people living with disability—and indeed, everyone."[8]

Types of Dementia

When I give talks about dementia-inclusive communities, one of the most common questions I hear is, "What is the difference between Alzheimer's and dementia?" (*Note: Readers who are already familiar with the difference, and with the most common types of dementia, may want to skip this section.*)

This question probably arises because of frequent references to "Alzheimer's and dementia" in popular media and public-policy statements by people who ought to know better. This makes it sound as if Alzheimer's and dementia are two unique conditions. I do not recall ever hearing anyone affiliated with the media or public policy refer to "Alzheimer's disease and related dementias," let alone "AD/ADRD." Also, the differentiation of "Alzheimer's disease" from "Alzheimer's dementia" described in Chapter 1 has been slow to catch on in public discourse.

A common metaphor for the term "dementia" is an umbrella under which one finds many specific diagnoses that present with a variety of cognitive, emotional, and behavioral changes. That slide my husband and I showed in 2013 had a drawing of an umbrella opened above a list of various types of dementia.

Dementia is a general category describing changes in the brain over time that can produce *cognitive* problems such as troubles with memory, problem-solving, decision-making, judgment, orientation to time and space, and language; difficulties with *emotion* regulation; and *motivational* challenges of goal-setting and determining the steps needed to accomplish a goal. All of these can be expressed through changes in people's actions. Some types of dementia do not initially present with memory problems. For example, with frontotemporal dementia, changes in personality occur initially without memory problems, such that an ordinarily easy-going person might become highly anxious or a kind person might start saying unkind things to loved ones.

It is important to state that some conditions that look like dementia are actually reversible. For example, in older people depression is sometimes described as "pseudo-dementia" because the depression amplifies their negative evaluation of their memory and their withdrawal from social contact. This is why a thorough diagnostic evaluation is so important. Other conditions, such as drug and alcohol abuse, adverse reactions to certain drugs, and normal pressure hydrocephalus, can produce dementia-like symptoms and can be treated.

Returning to the question about dementia and Alzheimer's, Alzheimer's dementia has traditionally been thought of as one specific type of dementia, and it is the most common dementia diagnosis, presently accounting for 60 to 80 percent of cases. Most of the time, Alzheimer's dementia emerges when people are in their late 60s and 70s, but as in the case of Peter Berry, who was introduced in Chapter 1, younger-onset Alzheimer's (also called "early-onset" Alzheimer's) dementia starts in midlife and sometimes earlier. Affecting about 5 percent of people diagnosed with Alzheimer's dementia, this condition has been definitively associated with particular genetic mutations and can be referred to as "familial Alzheimer's." Researchers have identified three rare genes that cause it.

Individuals living with younger-onset dementia in the United Kingdom organized a virtual community 20 years ago to offer support for one another and for families dealing with a condition that affects individuals still raising young children and participating in the workforce. This group now reaches people around the world through its website and newsletter. It includes those who have the familial type of Alzheimer's as well as other types of dementia described later in this chapter that can start when people are still relatively young.[9]

Many people wonder whether the common form of Alzheimer's dementia expressed in later life is inherited, and whether they should seek genetic testing. Several genes have been identified that can make a person more susceptible to developing late-onset Alzheimer's dementia. That susceptibility increases if a person inherits the risky gene from each parent. The issue of genetic testing for Alzheimer's dementia is complicated by the fact that, to date, no medications exist to cure or prevent the development of this form of dementia. However, some people choose to find out if they carry the genes associated either with familial or ordinary Alzheimer's dementia so they can actively pursue lifestyle changes in diet, exercise, cognitive stimulation, and social engagement that may reduce their risk or delay the onset of symptoms.

Although Alzheimer's dementia is by far the most common

dementia diagnosis, increasingly it is recognized that people can have "mixed dementia." Most often, the mix involves vascular dementia and Alzheimer's dementia.

Vascular dementia usually results from a series of small strokes that interfere with blood supply to the brain. Sometimes, vascular dementia occurs due to factors other than strokes, such as hypertension, that affect the brain's blood flow. Smoking, diabetes, and high cholesterol may also contribute to the development of vascular dementia, giving support to the statement that "what's good for the heart is good for the brain."[10] Vascular dementia does not necessarily become obvious because of memory impairment. Rather, a person might have problems with planning, organizing information, judgment, and making decisions. Clinicians often refer to these cognitive symptoms as revealing problems with executive function.

One can find conflicting statements in the scientific literature on the prevalence of the other dementias besides Alzheimer's dementia. Some say that vascular dementia is the next most prevalent disorder, but others claim that dementia with Lewy bodies (DLB) is next in line after Alzheimer's dementia.[11] This is probably of concern only to researchers and public-policy experts, especially since individuals can have more than one type of dementia.

DLB is most often characterized as presenting people with the challenge of vivid visual hallucinations, Parkinsonian-type movements, and physical actions when a person is dreaming. Symptoms often fluctuate during the day such that an individual might appear to be fine in one moment but then have speech problems and abrupt changes in attention (sometimes described as "zoning out").

Another type of dementia is frontotemporal dementia (FTD), a variant of which affected the woman with whom we spoke at the Minnesota conference. FTD may be noted first with personality changes such as a person becoming more impulsive and saying things she never would have uttered before the changes in the brain began (due to effects on the frontal lobes). It can also present primarily as problems with understanding language or in producing language (due to effects on the temporal lobes). The National Institute on Aging offers a good description of types of FTD on its website.[12]

I should note here that, although I refer in this book to "dementia-friendly and inclusive communities," a time may be coming when the word "dementia" disappears from the common lexicon. The most recent edition of the *Diagnostic and Statistical Manual* (DSM-5) of the American Psychiatric Association introduces the category of "neurocognitive disorders" (abbreviated as NCDs) and states that eventually it will replace "dementia" as an umbrella descriptor.[13] In the next chapter, I will address how the language we use to talk about the dementias can reinforce dementia stigma. Although it may be easier to say "the NCDs" and to describe someone as having "an NCD," this more scientific-sounding term has as much potential to convey the weight of stigma as the word "dementia" does currently.

NCDs can be major or mild, depending on the severity of symptoms. A mild NCD does not interfere with the ability to conduct ordinary life activities independently. However, the individual or a family member may start noting changes, including problems with memory, planning and multitasking, language (such as word-finding problems), and recognizing and responding appropriately to social cues such as other people's facial expressions. Depending on the type of dementia, when the NCD is mild, certain changes may raise concerns of the individuals experiencing them, family members, or friends. Typical responses would be to rationalize the changes as being due to aging itself or to simply ignore the changes. Those who have heard public-health messages about the importance of early diagnosis might encourage consultation with a physician. The line between a mild NCD and a major NCD will vary due to factors ranging from the individual's personal history to the social network surrounding the person. Progression to a major NCD produces significant, noticeable changes that interfere with the ability to carry out the ordinary tasks of everyday life. Examples include meal planning and preparation, maintaining a checking account, keeping track of appointments, driving, and way-finding.

Currently, the DSM-5 lists six other NCDs in addition to Alzheimer's, vascular, Lewy body, and frontotemporal dementia. In the coming years, many more may be added to the list. Already, subtypes of various NCDs have been identified.

The Problem of Progression

One of the defining characteristics of any of the dementias is that they are progressive conditions. Naturally, when people finally get a diagnosis (if they get one), they want to know how far along they are in the progression. We have become used to hearing about stages of cancer, and that is often one of the first questions family members and friends ask when they hear of someone's cancer diagnosis. The same is true for the dementias. Upon receiving a dementia diagnosis, it is natural to wonder what the future holds. Various stage models have been proposed, but like any stage model, they can be too rigidly applied, with little consideration of individual differences.

As described in Chapter 1, the NIA/AA guidelines introduced in 2011 differentiate three phases in the Alzheimer's disease process: the preclinical phase (no obvious symptoms), the mild-cognitive-impairment phase (when people have more problems with memory and other cognitive skills than most people their age), and the dementia phase (when clinical signs of Alzheimer's dementia become obvious). The first and most controversial phase is the asymptomatic preclinical phase that some researchers state can be detected through biomarkers such as analysis of accumulation of particular proteins—amyloid beta and tau—in cerebrospinal fluid or from images from PET scans or MRIs that show neuronal degeneration or injury. Most people do not have tests for these biomarkers unless they are enrolled in a research study, and the association of these biomarkers with Alzheimer's disease before symptoms emerge remains in question.

Earlier, I mentioned Dr. Ronald Petersen of Mayo Clinic, who gave the talk at the conference in Minnesota. His work on mild cognitive impairment launched a number of research efforts and elicited push-back from people concerned that a medical label was being attached to normal cognitive aging. Dr. Petersen always asserted that MCI is more than normal age-related forgetfulness and that people with MCI can continue most of the usual tasks of their lives. Controversy quickly arose in the first decade of this century when MCI became more widely discussed, with the controversy intensifying after 2011 when the NIA/AA diagnostic guidelines appeared.[14]

Researchers have reported conflicting evidence about the percentage of people who eventually experience some form of dementia after showing signs of memory problems (also called "amnestic" MCI) or problems with language, attention, visual perception, or figuring out the steps needed to do something ("non-amnestic" MCI). They call this the issue of conversion, as in converting from MCI to Alzheimer's dementia.

Some researchers claim that all persons with MCI eventually convert to Alzheimer's. Others report that some people get better on their own and that some learn to live with their MCI challenges with few signs of worsening. However, there is also good evidence showing that for many people MCI does eventually worsen, propelling them into the category of a dementia. Outside of the research laboratory, clinicians face the challenge of determining whether a patient's MCI symptoms could be due to a reversible, treatable condition or to a type of dementia for which pharmacologic treatments may only be effective early in the progression.[15] Some of these treatments are well known to people whose loved ones have received a diagnosis of Alzheimer's dementia. They include donepezil (Aricept) and memantine (Namenda), which are often prescribed together in an effort to slow the progression of symptoms.

The issue of progression is complex and depends upon the type of dementia as well as individual differences in physical, mental, and social health. Family members and close friends will often observe that things have changed over the course of years, months, and sometimes even days. Some people's dementia symptoms progress slowly and steadily, while others experience alternating plateaus and rapid declines. The person's clinician should be able to assess and describe the changes in a way that is helpful for planning. This is why it is important for people to return to their clinicians regularly, although for many reasons (such as costs, availability of clinicians, and denial by the person or family) this may not happen.

Diagnosing a Dementia

In nearly all the literature on dementia-friendly communities, one finds lists of defining characteristics, with most starting with "access to early diagnosis." This is, of course, easier said than done, since many people have no access to clinicians who specialize in dementia diagnosis. Nevertheless, organizations like Alzheimer's Disease International (ADI) have argued that it is a basic human right for people concerned about their cognitive well-being to receive a thorough, accurate diagnosis as soon as they start experiencing problems with the tasks of everyday life that could reflect the onset of a dementia. ADI acknowledges that even in high-income countries, up to half of all persons with a dementia never receive a diagnosis. The situation is much worse in low- and middle-income countries. In the United States, Latino and African American elders are less likely to receive a diagnosis for a number of reasons, including lack of access to health care and cultural beliefs about aging.

The World Alzheimer Report issued by ADI in 2011 stated that early diagnosis enables people to begin certain drug treatments that might slow symptom progression. Beyond drug therapies (which are not always effective and are not appropriate for all types of dementia), people need practical information about how they can live as well as possible with dementia symptoms.[16] Hopefully their clinicians will be aware of research showing how improvements in diet, exercise, mental stimulation, and social connectedness may help slow the progression and improve life quality.[17]

Unfortunately, some doctors are reluctant to give a dementia diagnosis even if they have a high degree of certainty resulting from examination of biomarkers and administration of cognitive tests of memory and thinking processes. They may assume that disclosure of the diagnosis would result in a "catastrophic emotional reaction," but this has not been shown to be common. In fact, research has shown that people are often relieved to have an explanation of their symptoms.[18] Without ever receiving a diagnosis, but with some recognition that she was struggling with memory and confusion, my mother used to joke that she had "Parts-heimer's disease." She claimed that her friends all said the same thing, indicating that they knew they had some problems but denied they could be due to Alzheimer's disease. How I wish she might have had a physician who did one of the brief cognitive screens now mandated for Medicare annual wellness checks. I am fairly certain she would not have been able to remember "apple, pencil, table" five minutes after her doctor first asked her to repeat those words. I suspect that she would have been one of the people having a catastrophic emotional reaction, but getting a diagnosis might have saved her considerable suffering at the end of her life. Because she had great social skills and could put on a good act at her doctor's office, no one ever suggested that she should be tested. Over the years, I have heard many stories similar to my mom's.

It doesn't have to be this way. People who are concerned about changes in cognition, emotion, and motivation should try to get a professional diagnostic evaluation that includes an interview about medical history, review of medications, a neurological exam, mental status exam, lab tests of blood and urine, and possibly a brain scan and additional neuropsychological testing.[19] As noted by Dr. Benjamin Mast, a leading neuropsychologist, this intense diagnostic process should be guided by the conviction that dementia does not rob an individual of humanity. In other words, the clinician needs to affirm the personhood of the patient instead of merely focusing on a bundle of biomedical issues. Mast describes a whole-person approach to dementia assessment that addresses the fears of people with symptoms and the ones who love them. Also, Mast urges clinicians to document their patients' strengths as well as their deficits.[20]

Do They Know?

In addition to the question about whether there is a difference between Alzheimer's and dementia, another question I often hear when I give talks about dementia is, "Do people know something is wrong?" This is a complicated issue that is usually raised when I only have a few minutes left before people start heading for the door. The quick answer I give is that some people are aware and acknowledge that they have noticed changes. Others are aware that something has changed but refuse to admit that they are aware, or they make excuses such as "I'm just not paying attention" (a statement I often heard my mother make). Finally, some people have little to no awareness, although their family members and friends may have noted numerous cognitive, emotional, and motivational problems. Sometimes that lack of awareness is an additional cause for concern because the neurological changes of dementia can affect awareness.

Awareness can also depend on how much the dementia has progressed. The person who has taught me the most about this complicated question of awareness is Dr. Linda Clare, a British neuropsychologist. She has studied awareness in people in the early stages of dementia still living independently as well as in people with severe dementia living in long-term care residences. With her colleagues, she has proposed four levels of awareness.

People with severe dementia can retain sensory awareness of stimuli in their environments. This is a crucial piece of information for those who care for them.[21] Even when these individuals have lost the ability to use language, they can demonstrate this level of awareness ("sensory registration") through movements and vocalization. Others, whose dementia has not progressed so much, are also aware of how well they are or are not performing various tasks ("performance monitoring"). In the early stage of dementia, people can describe the changes they are experiencing, something Dr. Clare and her colleagues call "evaluative judgment." Finally, some individuals in the early stage can reflect self-critically on these changes and the ways they affect their sense of themselves and their relationships with others ("meta-representation"). For people in the early stage, awareness interacts with the ways they cope with having a type of dementia. Some people try to make changes to adjust to their new reality, while others try to maintain life as it has always been.[22]

After the Diagnosis

Even if persons with dementia are aware of changes and agree to go through a multi-step diagnostic process, outcomes may be very different. Some people describe how their physician declared a diagnosis of Alzheimer's disease, prescribed some medications, gave them brochures from the Alzheimer's Association (or Alzheimer's Society), and basically said, "Good luck." I have also talked with people who went to highly respected medical clinics where they were told they might have "a little dementia." Others have related stories about doctors who said, "Everyone your age forgets things."

More fortunate people also learn about community programs and services designed to enable people with dementia to live as well as possible. This approach, called "social prescribing," is gaining attention from clinicians and researchers. Many of them are just as disappointed as people living with dementia that no breakthrough medications have been discovered in the search for a cure, or at least a guaranteed way to slow or even reverse symptom progression. Social prescribing is receiving support, especially in the UK and Canada, where people given a dementia diagnosis are encouraged to participate in arts programs, join exercise groups, visit museums, meditate, and do other activities that research has shown to be helpful in slowing dementia progression and improving life quality. For the person and care partner hearing the diagnosis, hope or hopelessness can be an outcome of how the diagnosis is delivered. It can also depend on having a clinician who understands the relationship between health care and social care. The clinician can provide health care, but social care happens in communities that strive to eliminate dementia stigma and provide opportunities for continued community engagement.

Whether a person holds on to hope or plunges into despair will also depend on numerous individual differences. These include age, financial security, personality, social networks, and sources of life meaning. The responses of family members and friends will also be a major influence. Some will try to deny the diagnosis by saying, "We all forget stuff" and "You don't look like you have dementia." Many people with dementia experience these types of responses as highly insulting. Others will ask "What stage are you in?" thinking that will provide some kind of definitive roadmap of the future. Richard Taylor, a clinical psychologist and author who received a diagnosis of "dementia, probably of the Alzheimer's type," often summarized the importance of recognizing individual differences in his speeches by offering a common observation, "When you've met one person with dementia, you've met one person with one form of dementia." Taylor might have added that you have met one person today whose dementia may be expressed differently the next time you meet because of the progressive nature of the condition.

So what is left? Is the situation hopeless? No! Eventually researchers may identify affordable pharmacological and other biomedical treatments that eliminate the symptoms of all types of dementia, but that outcome does not appear to be on the horizon for the next few decades. With no such medical treatments currently available, a different approach is needed, one that relies on the people living in our communities making the effort to offer programs and services to enrich the lives of everyone living with dementia.

With some education and inspiration, the usual view of dementia can be disrupted with a new story—a story about communities that offer hope through the preservation of dignity and meaningful relationships. A good place to begin is with the brief historical overview offered in the next chapter describing how thinking about dementia has evolved from the nineteenth century to the present.

Endnotes

1   I heard Dr. Miller use this term in a plenary talk he gave at the meeting of the Wisconsin Network Conference of the Alzheimer's Association in 2012. He said this trend began in the 1980s. In his talk he explained how people with frontotemporal dementia used to be misdiagnosed as having bipolar disorder or a personality disorder.

2   US Department of Health and Human Services. (2012). *National Plan to Address Alzheimer's Disease*. Washington, DC: US Department of Health and Human Services. Accessed on 7/12/19 at https://aspe.hhs.gov/system/files/pdf/102526/NatlPlan2012%20with%20Note.pdf

3   US Department of Health and Human Services. (2018). *National Plan to Address Alzheimer's Disease 2018 update*. Washington, DC: US Department of Health and Human Services. Accessed on 7/12/19 at https://aspe.hhs.gov/system/files/pdf/259581/NatPlan2018.pdf

4   Throughout the UK plan, one finds many engaging color photographs of people living with a dementia. No photos appear in the US plan.
     Department of Health. (2009). *Living well with dementia: A national dementia strategy*. London, UK: Department of Health, p. 3. Accessed on 7/12/19 at https://assets.publishing.service.gov.uk/government/uploads/system/uploads/attachment_data/file/168220/dh_094051.pdf

5   I first became aware of the importance of the words "the" and "a" when I read an article about creativity research and theory related to dementia. The authors referred to "the dementias" throughout the paper and talked about "people living with a dementia." In all my years of reading about dementia, I had never seen this. The paper lists 13 authors; all are associated with the Created Out of Mind Team in London (www.createdoutofmind.org). This is a consortium of persons having a dementia, scientists, and artists who, according to their website, are seeking to understand "art, consciousness, and the brain" by studying experiences of people living with a dementia.
     Camic, P. M., Crutch, S. J., Murphy, C., Firth, N. C., Harding, E., Harrison, C. R., et al. (2018). Conceptualising and understanding artistic creativity in the dementias: Interdisciplinary approaches to research and practise. *Frontiers in Psychology, 9*, 1–12.

6   Shakespeare, T., Zeilig, H., & Mittler, P. (2019). Rights in mind: Thinking differently about dementia and disability. *Dementia, 18*, 1075–1088. (p. 1083)

7   Shakespeare et al., pp. 1083–1084.

8   Shakespeare et al., p. 1085.

9   For more information about younger-onset dementia, as well as links to a network of people living with it, see www.youngdementiauk.org/about-us

10   Internet searches quickly identify many articles on all the dementias. However, one needs to be cautious in selecting ones that are legitimate and scientifically sound. See, for example, the website for Mayo Clinic; it offers a succinct description of types of vascular dementia: www.mayoclinic.org/diseases-conditions/vascular-dementia/symptoms-causes/syc-20378793

11   Adding to the confusion over types of dementias, some experts refer to "Dementia with Lewy bodies or DLB" while others discuss "Lewy body dementia or LBD." They are the same. The National Institute on Aging prefers the latter: www.nia.nih.gov/health/what-lewy-body-dementia

12   www.nia.nih.gov/health/types-frontotemporal-disorders

13   Most public libraries should have a copy of the DSM-5. The section on NCDs is well organized and easy to follow. It begins with a general description of mild and major NCDs and then gives diagnostic criteria for Alzheimer's dementia, frontotemporal lobar degeneration, Lewy body disease, vascular disease, and NCDs caused by brain injuries, medications, substances, toxins, infections, and other medical conditions such as multiple sclerosis, Huntington's disease, and endocrine diseases such as diabetes mellitus. For each category, the DSM-5 describes diagnostic features, prevalence, development and progression, risk factors, functional consequences, differential diagnosis (meaning how a clinician differentiates one condition from another), and comorbidity (other medical conditions that can complicate the picture).

     American Psychiatric Association. (2013). *Diagnostic and statistical manual of mental disorders* (5th ed.). Washington, DC: American Psychiatric Publishing.

     Also, the website of the Alzheimer's Association has a list of the most common forms of dementia, with links to more information about each one: www.alz.org/alzheimers-dementia/what-is-dementia/types-of-dementia

14   A paper published the year after the NIA/AA guidelines assessed their social and historical context in terms of the way we currently understand the brain and the humans who live with various brain changes labeled as diseases: George, D. R., Qualls, S. H., Camp, C. J., & Whitehouse, P. J. (2012). Renovating Alzheimer's: "Constructive" reflections on the new clinical and research diagnostic guidelines. *The Gerontologist, 53,* 378–387.

15   This question about the type of dementia is another reminder of the difference between the Alzheimer's-centric focus in the US and the broader approach taken in the UK. A guideline published in the UK by the National Institute for Health and Care Excellence begins by discussing how people vary—in other words, their individual differences—and argues that clinicians need to pay attention to "the human value of people living with dementia and their families and carers" as well as "how their personality and life experiences influence their response to dementia." The guideline helpfully recommends specific tests clinicians should use to differentiate different types of dementia and to decide what kinds of treatments to prescribe. See www.nice.org.uk/guidance/ng97

16   Prince, M., Bryce, R., and Ferri, C. (2011). *World Alzheimer Report 2011: The benefits of early diagnosis and intervention.* London, UK: Alzheimer's Disease International. Accessed on 7/13/19 at www.alz.co.uk/research/WorldAlzheimerReport2011.pdf

17   Hussenoeder, F. S., & Riedel-Heller, S. G. (2018). Primary prevention of dementia: From modifiable risk factors to a public brain health agenda? *Social Psychiatry and Psychiatric Epidemiology, 53,* 1280–1301.

18 Carpenter, B. D., Xiong, C., Porensky, E. K., Lee, M. M., Brown, P. J., Coats, M., et al. (2008). Reaction to a dementia diagnosis in individuals with Alzheimer's disease and mild cognitive impairment. *Journal of the American Geriatrics Society,* *56,* 401–412. (p. 405)

19 Many books and articles describe the different types of dementia, including those that may be reversible with medical treatment. One excellent resource, written by a compassionate geriatric psychiatrist, is written specifically for people caring for a loved one with dementia: Agronin, M. E. (2016). *The dementia caregiver: A guide to caring for someone with Alzheimer's disease and other neurocognitive disorders.* Lanham, MD: Rowman & Littlefield.

20 In my opinion, every clinician whose practice includes diagnosing dementias should read Mast's book: Mast, B. T. (2011). *Whole person dementia assessment.* Baltimore, MD: Health Professions Press.

21 Dr. Clare and her colleagues have developed a measure of awareness and have shown that when used by long-term-care staff, quality of life improves for residents because staff members realize that they are aware of their surroundings: Clare, L., Whitaker, R., Quinn, C., Jelley, H., Hoare, Z., Woods, B., et al. (2013). AwareCare: Development and validation of an observational measure of awareness in people with severe dementia. *Neuropsychological Rehabilitation: An International Journal,* *21*(1), 113–133.

22 Dr. Clare and her colleagues interviewed people in the early stages of Alzheimer's dementia about their awareness and the ways they cope. Quotes from these interviews reveal how people's sense of self is affected by the cognitive changes they are experiencing, their relationships with other people, and their own beliefs and personal coping resources: Clare, L., Roth, I., & Pratt, R. (2005). Perceptions of change over time in early-stage Alzheimer's disease. *Dementia, 4,* 487–520.

Chapter 3

From Senility and Stigma to Citizenship

Sometimes it's necessary to go a long distance out of the way in order to come back a short distance correctly.

—Edward Albee, *The Zoo Story*[1]

In July 2006, I had the great pleasure of lounging for a few days beside a swimming pool at a small hotel in San Leonino, Italy, a tiny village near Siena. Adding to the wonder of that time was my immersion in a book by historian Jesse Ballenger called *Self, Senility, and Alzheimer's Disease in Modern America: A History*.[2] At times, though, I felt as if I should have wrapped plain brown paper around the book's cover. I figured that anyone who could read English might think that my vacation-book selection was strange. Then I recognized that feeling as a sign itself of the pervasiveness of dementia stigma, all because of one word in the book's title: "senility."

Although I have been thinking about dementia for several decades, I have rarely considered the meaning of senility. It always seemed like both an old-fashioned word and a pejorative image attached to older people. However, a few years ago, the title of a journal article in a reference list popped out at me. Appearing in 1978, the article was called "The Senile Dement in Our Midst: A Look at the Other Side of the Coin."[3] Immediately I found that language off-putting. Senile dement? I'd never heard of such a label. Naturally, I had to track down the article.

The author, Dr. Frances Hellebrandt, was "a woman pioneer in exercise physiology, physical medicine, and rehabilitation" who taught at the University of Wisconsin–Madison.[4] After she retired in 1964, she moved to First Community Village outside of Columbus, Ohio, which was one of the first continuum-of-care retirement communities in the country. There she continued to write professional papers, including the one I read. She described people with "senile dementia" living comfortably "in the midst of the unaffected."[5] However, when their wandering and disorientation threatened their safety, staff relocated them to the secure Convalarium, the skilled nursing wing. Dr. Hellebrandt regularly visited that area and observed the staff's "respect for the senile dement as an individual."[6] She said that staff focused on residents' strengths, not their losses. She also described residents' ability to display "astonishingly adept social manners"[7] and told how they enjoyed various group activities. She concluded by saying that she was an unusual "villager" for venturing into the Convalarium, observing that the "idea of age-related disability is repugnant, especially if the disability involves intellectual competence."[8] Her final paragraph began with this plea: "We must treat the senile dements in our midst as adults."[9]

Dr. Hellebrandt died at First Community Village in 1992. As if her gentle observations were not enough to elicit my appreciation of her paper, learning about her life amplified my feelings about her. Also, my mother died at the same First Community Village in 2013, just as she was about to be transferred to the secure memory-care area, now called The Roxbury Cottages.

The word "senility" seems to have largely disappeared from most people's vocabularies, although it still occasionally pops up in unusual places. For example, this headline appeared in 2015: "9th Circuit Addresses Senility Among Federal Judges Head On."[10] A widely distributed news release described how the Ninth Circuit Court of Appeals (California and eight other Western states) was educating its justices (who serve with life tenure) about cognitive changes associated with dementia.

Cognitive changes due to some type of dementia are a legitimate concern not just for families and friends but also for all types of organizations, including, of course, the judiciary. Some justices are appointed for life, which means that they can still be serving in their 80s and 90s when the risk of dementia is high merely due to age.

Aside from the surprising use of the word "senility" in that article, I was glad to know that the court was addressing the risk of a judge showing signs of dementia while making life and death decisions.

As more people live longer, sometimes work longer, and also receive a dementia diagnosis, families, communities, professional organizations, and governing bodies will need to engage in difficult conversations about what Dr. G. Allen Power calls "negotiated risk."[11] Can Grandma still use her stove? Can Grandpa keep his guns? When should my friend stop driving? Is it okay for that nursing-home resident to take a walk in the neighborhood? Can that professor continue to teach? Can the surgeon still operate?[12]

Questions like these likely never arose when we used to call someone senile simply because that person was old. But then, from the end of the nineteenth century (when life expectancy in the United States was 47 years) to the present, many social beliefs about aging and dementia changed. Twentieth-century medical triumphs such as antibiotics and reductions in infant mortality among some populations produced a remarkable increase in life expectancy by the end of the century. At the same time, the population bulge produced by the baby-boom cohort born between 1946 and 1964 brought the dawning realization that all those babies would someday be old and could possibly develop a dementia. With predictions of burgeoning numbers of older people, the issue of how much risk societies could tolerate became more pressing.

Although we no longer mockingly label people living with a dementia as senile, considerable stigma remains attached to their condition. However, with more people telling a new story about dementia, some cracks are appearing in that wall of stigma that separates people living with dementia from their communities. To better understand the call for dementia-inclusive and friendly communities, including debates about how much risk can be tolerated by these communities, we need to pause and ask how we got here. In other words, as the epigraph for this chapter suggests, sometimes you have to go a long way out of your way to gain a better understanding of where you are now.

Age and Dementia; Ageism and "Dementism"

When I give talks introducing audiences to basic information about dementia, I often show one slide that illustrates the arc of the dementia story and use of the word "senility" from the nineteenth century through the present day. Early in the nineteenth century, someone like Thomas Jefferson could talk about looking forward to retirement when he could play with his grandchildren and enjoy "senile rest." But by the end of that century, senility had acquired a pejorative association with older people and with both physical and mental decline.[13] At the beginning of the twentieth century, physicians employed labels such as "organic brain syndrome" and "senile psychosis" in clinical descriptions of older persons with memory problems. By the 1980s, a disease-specific, eponymous term became more widely employed: "Alzheimer's disease."

The story of how we got from senility to Alzheimer's disease is a fascinating tale of politics, medicine, and research. The story takes place in the context of dramatic changes in attitudes about aging, old age, and older adults—the three areas addressed by the field of gerontology that emerged at the end of World War II. Thomas Cole, a professor of medical humanities, illustrated these changes in his 1992 book *The Journey of Life* by including reproductions of images created to portray the ages (or stages) of life beginning in the eleventh century when the journey was represented by a circle or a wheel (hence the origin of the phrase "wheel of fortune"). Over the course of many centuries, there was no linear representation of a beginning (birth) or end (death) of life. Rather, as Cole stated, "all time belonged to God."[14]

The circle broke in the sixteenth century with the emergence of images of the ages of life portrayed as a climb up an arched bridge from birth to midlife power and prosperity (for men, not women) and then a descent to decrepitude and death. Religious exhortations about sin and repentance and about damnation and salvation appeared under the bridge's arch. The placement of these religious images symbolically communicated that they applied to all parts of the life span.

By the nineteenth century, religious references disappeared completely in some stages-of-life illustrations. For example, in 1836 a print depicting the "life and age of woman" showed a mother instructing her daughter under the arch and saying "the virtuous woman is a crown to her husband." And then the famous printers Currier and Ives jumped on the bandwagon around 1850 by producing stages-of-life illustrations for men (notably with a woman caring for a dying man), for women (shown dying alone), and for drunkards.[15]

Cole argued that ageism—prejudice and discrimination against people based solely on advanced age—began in the late nineteenth century with the fading influence of Calvinist assertions that all people's lives mix loss and gain as well as sin and redemption.[16] Individuals were viewed either as virtuous by dint of their own hard work and self-discipline (for example, with their habits of eating, drinking, earning, and saving money) or as society's dregs whose diseases, poverty, and dependence derived from their unwillingness to work hard and take care of themselves and their families. Older people could fall into either category, but those who showed signs of physical or mental frailty were seen as having failed to live a morally disciplined life. In other words, their frailty was their fault. This devaluing of elderhood coincided with political changes that emphasized fresh, new, youthful leadership rather than the wisdom and experience offered by many older people.

In his 2006 book about the history of self, senility, and Alzheimer's disease, Jesse Ballenger touched on themes that are similar to the ones raised by Cole. He agreed that by the end of the nineteenth century in the US good health was seen as a reward for a life lived well according to the moral values espoused by the American evangelical religion of the times. Signs of senile dementia indicated that a person had failed to live a virtuous life and had depleted the vital energy present at birth. This meant that now people not only dreaded suffering the loss of mental acuity in old age but also dreaded what that meant in terms of their foundation of selfhood. People were seen as responsible for creating their own healthy selfhood through hard work and moral commitments. However, selfhood could disappear with the onset of senility. As Ballenger aptly stated, "senility haunts the landscape of the self-made man."[17]

The story of fear and stigma attached to old age and dementia became even more complicated in the mid-twentieth century with the birth of gerontology as a specific, multidisciplinary field of study.

Gerontologists sought to fight the good fight against ageism, lifting up images of successful elders who were healthy, mentally sharp, and meaningfully engaged with the world. Unfortunately, all of this hopeful talk about older people's vitality left the impression that those who lacked that vitality, whether physically or mentally, had somehow failed at aging. As I mentioned earlier, this meant that older people were split into two categories: those who were aging well and contradicting ageist assumptions, and those who were not.[18]

According to ethicist Stephen Post, this splitting of well elders from ill elders produced "dementism": prejudice and discrimination against persons having a dementia.[19] Post argued that equating mental acuity with moral superiority is evidence of the hypercognitive culture of the West going back to the Cartesian statement "I think, therefore I am." Although most deeply forgetful persons can still respond to objects, places, and people in ways that reflect emotional and relational connection, often they are not afforded dignity and respect for their remaining capacities because they have lost the cognitive abilities so highly valued in Western culture. Post's position on ethics and dementia derives from his observation that when cognition is given greater social value than feelings and relationality, people living with dementia risk being marginalized, abused, and neglected.

What's in a Name?

In 1906, Dr. Alois Alzheimer conducted an autopsy on the brain of Auguste D., a 57-year-old woman. She is famous for being the first person for which there is clinical and histological evidence of what we now call Alzheimer's disease. Dr. Alzheimer had begun caring for her five years earlier when she was admitted to a psychiatric clinic in Frankfurt, Germany, and so he was able to document the progression of her condition. His case reports of Auguste D. would sound familiar to physicians assessing patients with dementia today, for they showed how she struggled to recall words and to answer his questions. At one point in an interview with Dr. Alzheimer, she poignantly stated, "I have lost myself."[20]

In a paper published the year after Auguste D.'s death, Dr. Alzheimer described the amyloid plaques (outside the neurons) and the neurofibrillary tangles (inside the neurons) of her brain. Shortly after that publication, and another one describing a second case, a famous German psychiatrist named Dr. Emil Kraepelin gave Auguste D.'s condition a name: Alzheimer's disease. The reason he did this is still debated, but the bottom line for both Kraepelin and Alzheimer was that they now had possible evidence of the organic basis of this progressive loss of cognitive function.[21]

Soon, however, the question arose of whether what Dr. Alzheimer had observed in Auguste D.'s behavior and then in her brain was the same disease as senile dementia, a condition described by many nineteenth-century psychiatrists as occurring in older people. Kraepelin thought Auguste D.'s disease was different, a new disease that could be called "presenile dementia." Dr. Alzheimer disagreed, stating in a paper in 1911 that what he had observed in Auguste D. was not different from senile dementia and that all he had discovered was that it could occur in younger people. Thus, Dr. Alzheimer seemed to reject the attachment of his name to a new disease because he did not think it was actually new.

As told by Jesse Ballenger, the story of Alzheimer's disease resided in a kind of intellectual and clinical backwater of psychiatry through the early part of the 1900s. Debate over whether presenile and senile dementia were the same disease continued. Moreover, there were now findings that some older people have brains that appear to show pathological signs of Alzheimer's disease but thinking and behavior that show little clinical evidence of progressive loss of cognitive function. Also, this next question was being debated by the few researchers and clinicians paying attention to dementia: Was there a specific disease process occurring to produce the symptoms experienced by some people, or did those persons have the misfortune of displaying some kind of acceleration of the normal cognitive changes of aging?

These debates about dementia were not widely noted by American psychiatrists of the time, because many adopted the psychodynamic approach to mental disorders promoted by Freud and others. In other words, they were not so concerned with the biological underpinnings of the disorders they were treating. However, as the Freudian hold on American psychiatry loosened after World War II, and as biomedical models of psychiatric disorders became more widely accepted, interest in the underlying pathology of dementia grew, especially because some evidence pointed to deficits of a certain neurotransmitter (acetylcholine) that might be addressed pharmacologically.[22]

By the 1960s, senility as a normally occurring condition in old people had morphed into a disease defined by specific brain pathologies that might point toward ways to cure the disease, prevent it, or at least slow its progression. Now politics entered the scene, because a formerly obscure condition was starting to attract attention among people concerned about the demographics of aging. If more people were going to be living longer, and thus be susceptible to this disease, then a large amount of money would be needed for researchers trying to unlock its secrets and find ways to treat it.

In 1974, the US Congress approved the establishment of the National Institute on Aging (NIA), led initially by Dr. Robert Butler, a highly regarded geriatric psychiatrist. Since no one could argue that money was needed to "cure" aging, Dr. Butler knew the NIA could only attract scientific interest and political support by identifying a disease that could be addressed by this new institute within the National Institutes of Health.

A few years later, a group of researchers, physicians, and family caregivers established an organization called the Alzheimer's Disease and Related Disorders Association (ADRDA), which later shortened its name and narrowed its focus by becoming the Alzheimer's Association. Shortly afterwards, an argument broke out among the groups that formed the ADRDA, with some urging funding for care for persons having Alzheimer's disease and support for their caregivers. Others held out for money to fund basic research that might eventually produce a cure.[23]

Care or cure? This is an ongoing controversy, with both sides using what is sometimes called "apocalyptic demography" to support their positions.[24] Ballenger describes the fight over care versus cure as expressing the "politics of anguish." In the end, the argument that the scourge of polio had been eliminated through basic medical research tipped the balance toward research to find a cure. The anguish came not only from caregivers and people with dementia who felt that their needs were not being addressed but also from the frightening images used to support the need to fund basic research. These images were often cast in financial terms—as in, the aging baby-boom cohort will bankrupt world economies if no cure can be found.

Another consequence of apocalyptic demography and the politics of anguish was that people living with dementia were now viewed solely through the lens of disease that attacked their brains. Some authors even claimed that the disease robbed people of selfhood and represented a kind of death for a person left only as a hollow shell. These images may have motivated some people to donate to the Alzheimer's Association and other organizations raising funds for Alzheimer's research (although the effectiveness of fear as a motivational tactic to do good is questionable), but they also had the unintended consequence of further stigmatizing individuals having dementia.

The Story Shifts: From Senility and Brain Disease to Personhood and Social Citizenship

Dr. Alzheimer died in 1915, so he could not have known how the presenile dementia he identified in Auguste D. would be described at the end of the twentieth century as a worldwide "epidemic" bearing his name. He also could not have known that his name would be affixed to a "disease movement" with social and political forces shaping it.[25] In other words, this is not merely a story about brains having the amyloid plaques and neurofibrillary tangles he identified. It is a story about human beings contending with beliefs about their condition that define them as having a frightening brain disease for which money must be raised to find a cure. As we will see in Chapters 4 and 5, people living with dementia in many parts of the world are resisting that narrow definition by insisting on their rights as full persons to remain included within their communities.

The new story about dementia being written now builds on themes expressed toward the end of the last century. As I mentioned earlier, an important shift occurred with the publication of Tom Kitwood's 1997 book *Dementia Reconsidered: The Person Comes First*. Kitwood critiqued the biomedical model of dementia that prioritized discussions of diseased brains. He called for a new way of thinking about people living with dementia that emphasized personhood. He famously defined personhood as a standing or status that is bestowed upon one human being by others in the context of particular social relationships and institutional arrangements. It implies recognition, respect, and trust.[26]

In other words, personhood implies relationships. The experience of dementia is not merely shaped by what happens in an individual's brain. The neurological changes are certainly important, but they need to be viewed within the context of a complex, dynamic interaction of that person's personality, life history, physical health, and social connections.

Kitwood's book awakened people's imaginations about how the dementia story might shift from fatalism about brain deterioration to hopeful support for meaningful social relationships regardless of the type or severity of dementia. About a decade later, Ruth Bartlett and Deborah O'Connor wrote a book that moved discourse about dementia to what they described as the "fourth movement" in the story. As told by Bartlett and O'Connor, the story began with senility, moved to the biomedical emphasis on diseased brains, and then was transformed by Kitwood's vision of personhood as grounded in relationships. However, Bartlett and O'Connor argued that the story should not end there because it fails to account for the varied settings of people's lives. Personhood, they said, is located within particular interpersonal environments and sociocultural contexts. Thus, the fourth movement emphasizes "social citizenship," defined by Bartlett and O'Connor as

a relationship, practice or status in which a person with dementia is entitled to experience freedom from discrimination, and to have opportunities to grow and participate in life to the fullest extent possible. It involves justice, recognition of social positions, and the upholding of personhood, rights, and a fluid degree of responsibility for shaping events at a personal and societal level.[27]

Bartlett and O'Connor's writings about social citizenship lie behind much contemporary discussion of dementia-inclusive communities. Although some people might read their definition as applying only to people whose dementia has not progressed to the point where they have lost language, control over bodily functions, and the ability to live independently, Bartlett and O'Connor never meant to exclude them.

Applying Bartlett and O'Connor's ideas specifically to people living with advanced dementia in long-term-care settings, Canadian public-health scientist Pia Kontos and her colleagues have extended the model of social citizenship by emphasizing relationship-centered care and what they call "embodied selfhood."[28] That means that people who initially appear to be unable to interact deliberately with their environments through language or movement still can demonstrate selfhood and relationality in their individual preferences for people, sounds (especially music), gentle touch, sweet tastes, and calming scents.

Consider this example. Sue has lived in a memory-care community for several years as her dementia symptoms have become more severe. She can no longer control her body and balance enough to walk safely, so she uses a wheelchair that must be pushed by others. Staff who tend to her needs (including basic functions like eating, dressing, and using the bathroom) know her well. She rarely speaks and has trouble coordinating movement of her head. Nevertheless, anyone carefully observing interactions between Sue and staff can see that they share a meaningful relationship. When brought to an activity, Sue raises her head just enough to look at the person who has transported her and flashes a brief smile. She lifts her right hand slightly in a wave of acknowledgment. When someone kneels by her wheelchair and grasps her hands, she squeezes them. In other words, Sue is engaging with others—being relational—through her body.

To summarize this section with the help of Sue, consider that "once upon a time" she would have been dismissed as hopelessly senile. If her condition were defined as destruction of her brain (which, according to some, would make her less than human), she might have been warehoused and labeled as a hopeless burden on society. Fortunately, she lives today in an environment that respects her personhood. Although she cannot participate in the actions most often associated with social citizenship, which is defined by active roles and tasks in community, she can still give and receive the warmth and mutuality of relational citizenship. Sue is an important part of the small household and larger neighborhood of her memory-care community. Staff members comment that her flash of a smile and a wave can brighten their days. Despite her many limitations, Sue can still contribute to the well-being of others.

We've Come a Long Way

At the beginning of this chapter, I noted that we might have to go a long distance out of our way (namely by reviewing the history of Western attitudes about dementia) in order to understand the contemporary call for dementia-friendly and inclusive communities. Now we have some context for understanding some of the clearest evidence of changes in perspectives on dementia: we are slowly revising the way we talk about the condition and the people who live with it.

Here is another example. Although we rarely hear people labeled as senile these days, one scholar has documented multiple references in the dementia literature to "zombies" and the "walking dead."[29] Compared with those harsh descriptions, saying a person is engaging in "challenging" or "disruptive" behaviors may seem more benign. But we need to take a closer look at those terms, as well.

Often, people working in long-term-care communities use the word "behaviors" in reference to actions that are disruptive or challenging for them. Although "behavior" is a neutral term depicting any observable action, in the world of dementia care it has acquired a negative connotation. Much literature on so-called "behavioral and psychological symptoms of dementia" (also known as BPSDs) fails to recognize that a person's actions often represent attempts to communicate some kind of distress. Calling these actions "symptoms" invites a biomedical response with antipsychotic medication, even though clinical research shows little benefit and greater risk (including risk of death) from such medications.[30]

In Canada, there is a movement to use the term "responsive behaviors" to indicate that various actions, words, and gestures are expressions (often intentional) of distressing physical or cognitive issues. A person's actions could reflect pain; frustration about their ability to think and communicate; emotional vulnerability; a feeling of being unsettled by environmental stimuli; or a mismatch between what she can do and what she is being asked to do.[31] Redirecting long-term staff to consider what residents are attempting to communicate opens the way for a new formulation of BPSDs. Christine Bryden, an Australian writer and activist living with dementia, says that we should think of BPSDs as indicating "bio-psycho-social distress."[32]

Organizations working to create dementia-friendly communities in Australia, Ireland, and the United Kingdom have produced guides for changing the language used to talk about the condition of dementia and the people who live with it. Progress has been made, although one still hears people throughout the developed world refer to a demographic "silver tsunami" of older people at risk of developing dementia. Tsunamis kill people and wreak terrible damage on the environment. Dementia, and aging in general, should not be burdened with those images. Another harmful metaphor is the description of dementia prevalence as an "epidemic." What do we do when an epidemic strikes a community? We quarantine people, isolating them from healthy others in order to prevent the spread of contagion. Dementia is not contagious, and social isolation can contribute to worsening symptoms.

Similarly, because dementia has been narrowly conceptualized as a medical issue, people living with dementia are often called "dementia patients." The word "patient" should only be applied in a medical setting such as a clinic or a hospital. After all, many people have arthritis, but they probably do not want to be categorized as "arthritis patients" unless they are visiting their doctor. Even in that setting, more individuals today are insisting that they be viewed and treated as whole persons who happen to have painful knees or hips.

In 2015, the US-based Dementia Action Alliance (DAA) produced a helpful online publication called *Living Fully with Dementia: Words Matter*. It refuted what we all learned as children that although "sticks and stones" can harm us, names cannot. But they can! They can shape how people with dementia are treated, consequently affecting how they think and feel about themselves. Here is an example offered by Michael Ellenbogen (quoted in the DAA document), a man diagnosed with younger-onset Alzheimer's dementia at age 49, who began living with its symptoms when he was 39:

> I do not like the term "patient" unless I am in a hospital or medical setting. If I hear this word used to refer to me in other settings, it weakens me and I worry I will start acting like a patient and need someone to do even more for me.[33]

Even in a hospital or clinician's office, some language used today to talk about the dementias can be upsetting. For example, I recently became aware of how troubling the new term "neurocognitive disorder" (NCD) can be. This is especially true when the word "major" is affixed to NCD. A 68-year-old woman told me about how devastated she felt, for multiple reasons, being given the diagnosis of "major neurocognitive disorder due to Alzheimer's disease," including the fact that the descriptor "major" seemed to close all possibilities for hope. Not only was she upset about how the clinician revealed the diagnosis, she was also unhappy that she received no information about how she and her husband might cope with her major NCD. She described her county as a "dementia desert" with few resources for her as a diagnosed person or for him as a care partner.

I recently described this woman's response to my friend, Dr. Abhilash Desai, a geriatric psychiatrist in Idaho and author of many books and papers on the importance of person-centered medical care for people living with dementia.[34] I asked him about the language he uses when giving a diagnosis. He replied:

> Even before I begin an assessment, I tell the patient and family that I would like them to think about how they might react to certain words. If I say "dementia" or "Alzheimer's" or "major neurocognitive disorder" after I complete my assessment, how might they feel? Then we discuss what would be the best words to use, and I tell them, "Why even bother with a 'diagnosis' and labels and words. Let's just create a cognitive-emotional-spiritual wellness plan that includes correcting any reversible causes of cognitive decline." Many words nowadays have taken on such a toxic effect that, for many of my patients, I don't think they are worth the benefits!

Dr. Desai used to practice in the city where I live. He organized many small conferences to which he invited his patients, their care partners, health-care professionals, social workers, and others who worked with elders, especially those having dementia. I once heard him give a talk at one of these conferences in which he recommended ways of maintaining brain health regardless of whether a person has a dementia diagnosis. One older woman who attended the talk and was one of his patients living with dementia later told me she nearly skipped down the hall afterwards to tell him that he had given her back her life. She was not a "dementia patient," and certainly not a "senile dement" with a collection of symptoms. She was a person living with a dementia that did not prevent her from wanting to live as well as possible, without prejudice and discrimination, just like any other citizen in her community. Such is the power of words to convey a message of hope despite the many difficulties dementia brings to people's lives.[35]

People living with a dementia are speaking up to insist that their human rights be honored and that the dementia deserts be eliminated. These are individuals who have had multiple roles and responsibilities through adulthood in their communities. They want to continue to be treated with dignity and encouraged to remain hopeful despite the reality of dementia progression. Another way of saying this is that they do not want to lose the privileges of citizenship and opportunities to be helpful to others just because they have a dementia diagnosis. The next two chapters introduce several of these people and describe how they are speaking up not only for themselves but also for everyone living with a dementia diagnosis. Their experience illuminates a path for all of us.

Endnotes

1   Albee, E. (2008). *The zoo story*. New York, NY: William Morris Endeavor Entertainment, LLC. (Original work published 1959). Reproduced with kind permission from William Morris Endeavor Entertainment, LLC.

2   Ballenger, J. F. (2006). *Self, senility, and Alzheimer's disease in modern America: A history*. Baltimore, MD: Johns Hopkins University Press.

3   Hellebrandt, F. A. (1978). The senile dement in our midst: A look at the other side of the coin. *The Gerontologist, 18*(1), 67–70.

4   This memorial resolution for Dr. Hellebrandt (appearing 10 years after she died) is worth reading: Brown, J. (2002). *Memorial resolution of the faculty of the University of Wisconsin–Madison: On the death of Professor Emerita Frances A. Hellebrandt, M.D.* Madison, WI: University of Wisconsin–Madison, p. 1. Accessed on 7/13/19 at https://kb.wisc.edu/images/group222/shared/2002-10-07FacultySenate/1656(mem_res).pdf

5   Hellebrandt, p. 67.

6   Hellebrandt, p. 68.

7   Hellebrandt, p. 68.

8   Hellebrandt, p. 70.

9   Hellebrandt, p. 70.

10 Thanawala, S. (2015, November 7). *9th circuit addresses senility among federal judges head on*. Business Insider. Accessed on 7/16/19 at www.businessinsider.com/ap-9th-circuit-addresses-senility-among-federal-judges-head-on-2015-11

11 Power places negotiated risk in the context of liability concerns on one side and what he terms "the tendency toward surplus safety" on the other side. More detail about his ideas about negotiated risk and the need to honor the autonomy of persons having dementia appears in Chapter 8: Power, G. A. (2014). *Dementia beyond disease: Enhancing well-being*. Baltimore, MD: Health Professions Press.

12 The capacity of older physicians to provide high-quality health care of all kinds has been debated for a long time. Similar debates regarding mandatory retirement based on age alone have arisen in other professions (such as airline pilots) that concern public safety. A review of issues pertinent to the medical profession reported that 23 percent of practicing physicians in the US in 2015 were 65 or older: Dellinger, E. P., Pellegrini, C. A., & Gallagher, T. H. (2017). The aging physician and the medical profession: A review. *JAMA Surgery, 152*(10), 967–971.

13 Ballenger, p. 13.

14 This book is a notable example of how the disciplines of the humanities—history, philosophy, religious studies, art—can be interwoven to tell a fascinating story: Cole, T. R. (1992). *The journey of life: A cultural history of aging in America*. New York, NY: Cambridge University Press. (p. 15)

15 These images of arched bridges evolved into the hill metaphor and bad jokes about people who are "over the hill." A few years ago, a student presented me with a table decoration she got at a party store. I've taken it to many talks about ageism for "show and tell." It is a kind of fountain of thin, shiny plastic ribbons. Attached to many of the ribbons are cardboard squares announcing "Over the hill!" Attached to other ribbons are foil cut-outs with a number: 30. It always startles my audiences when they imagine a birthday party for someone turning 30 who is now viewed as being over the hill.

16 Dr. Robert Butler, founding director of the National Institute on Aging, coined the term "ageism" in an article describing opposition to a public-housing project for low-income older people. He observed that meetings about the project turned into a "middle-aged riot" by people who did not want old people, especially poor old people, living in their neighborhood: Butler, R. N. (1969). Age-ism: Another form of bigotry. *The Gerontologist, 9*, 243–246.

17 Ballenger, p. 9.

18 In 2003, Martha Holstein and Meredith Minkler published one of the most widely cited critiques of categorizing elders as "successful" as long as they were free of disease and disability, maintained physical and mental functioning, and remained engaged with life: Holstein, M. B., & Minkler, M. (2003). Self, society, and the "new gerontology." *The Gerontologist, 43*, 787–796.

An interview with Holstein 15 years later demonstrated how she connected this critique to a feminist analysis of social expectations for aging women: www.silvercentury.org/2018/03/martha-holstein-feminism-and-the-future-of-aging

19 Post, S. (2000). *The moral challenge of Alzheimer disease: Ethical issues from diagnosis to dying* (2nd ed.). Baltimore, MD: Johns Hopkins University Press.

20 It is fascinating to read Dr. Alzheimer's detailed clinical notes about Auguste D. in which he describes her symptoms and his interactions with her. Konrad Maurer and his colleagues have written several books and papers about Alzheimer's work and legacy; see, for example, Maurer, K., Volk, S., & Gerbaldo, H. (2000). Auguste D.: The history of Alois Alzheimer's first case. In P. J. Whitehouse, K. Maurer, & J. F. Ballenger (Eds.), *Concepts of Alzheimer disease: Biological, clinical, and cultural perspectives* (pp. 5–29). Baltimore, MD: Johns Hopkins University Press.

21 At the time of these publications, Freud's work was attracting considerable attention among psychiatrists. However, although Freud always contended that there would eventually be organic evidence for the symptoms he described, he did not have that evidence. Thus, Kraepelin could claim that his Munich laboratory was superior to Freud's Viennese couch.

22 This research led to the development of cholinesterase inhibitors that worked to increase levels of acetylcholine, reductions of which had been observed in people and animals with memory problems. The drugs developed through this research included tacrine (Cognex), donepezil (Aricept), and rivastigmine (Exelon).

23 As depicted in a recent article, this argument about imbalance in the "dual mission" of the Alzheimer's Association (support for care; support for cure) continues today: Caspi, E. (2019). Trust at stake: Is the "dual mission" of the US Alzheimer's Association out of balance? *Dementia, 18*, 1629–1650.

24 The first reference I can find to "apocalyptic demography" came in a paper arguing that the dread about Alzheimer's disease had been socially constructed in order to attract more government funding for research. Thus, we see a continuation of the argument begun in Dr. Alzheimer's time about whether Alzheimer's disease represented a specific disease category or was a variant on normal aging: Robertson, A. (1990). The politics of Alzheimer's disease: A case study in apocalyptic demography. *International Journal of Health Services, 20*(3), 429–442.

25 See this article by Patrick Fox for an early description of the Alzheimer's disease movement: Fox, P. (1989). From senility to Alzheimer's disease: The rise of the Alzheimer's disease movement. *The Milbank Quarterly, 67*, 58–102.

26 Kitwood, T. (1997). *Dementia reconsidered: The person comes first*. Philadelphia, PA: Open University Press. (p. 8)

27 Bartlett, R., & O'Connor, D. (2010). *Broadening the dementia debate: Towards social citizenship*. Portland, OR: Policy Press. (p. 37)

28 Kontos, P., Miller, K-L., & Kontos, A. P. (2017). Relational citizenship: Supporting embodied selfhood and relationality in dementia care. *Sociology of Health & Illness, 39*(2), 182–198.

29 Many journal articles are written with off-putting academic language, but this one is not. It is worth contacting a librarian to get a copy in order to read about the horrifying depictions of people living with dementia: Behuniak, S. M. (2011). The living dead? The construction of people with Alzheimer's disease as zombies. *Aging & Society, 31*, 70–92.

30 Desai, A. K., & Desai, F. G. (2014). Management of behavioral and psychological symptoms of dementia. *Current Geriatrics Reports, 3*(4), 259–272. (p. 264)

31 https://alzheimer.ca/en/on/We-can-help/Resources/Shifting-Focus/What-are-responsive-behaviours

32 Bryden's comment about renaming BPSDs appeared in a report produced by the Dementia Action Alliance. A summary of the report can be found here: https://daanow.org/wp-content/uploads/2020/05/WORDS-MATTER-Revisions.pdf

33 People living with dementia helped write the Dementia Action Alliance's report about language. It is a good example of abiding by this slogan from the disability rights movement: "nothing about us without us." See https://daanow.org/wp-content/uploads/2020/05/WORDS-MATTER-Revisions.pdf.

34 Dr. Desai and his colleague, Dr. George T. Grossberg, wrote a helpful book for people working in long-term-care settings. They included many case studies and wrote in a manner that is accessible for non-medically trained persons but is at the same time an accurate, thorough, evidence-based book for health-care

professionals: Desai, A. K., & Grossberg, G. T. (2017). *Psychiatric consultation in long-term care: A guide for health-care professionals* (2nd ed.). New York, NY: Cambridge University Press.

35 Dr. Desai believes in social prescribing. For example, when he practiced in my town, he got a small grant to hire a music therapist to conduct weekly sessions at his clinic. I attended several times and was astonished to observe people walking into a geriatric psychiatrist's office with smiles on their faces.

Part 2

HEARING THEIR VOICES

Chapter 4

People Living with Dementia Tell a New Story

President Ronald Reagan. Justice Sandra Day O'Connor. Glen Campbell. Sir Terry Pratchett. Pat Summitt. What do they have in common? Like many other famous people, their names appear on lists of well-known individuals with a dementia diagnosis. Unlike most of the others on those lists, soon after seeing their doctors they announced their diagnoses by publicly stating that they were living with a condition many people still try to hide.

This culture of secrecy includes the physicians of persons living with dementia. According to research by the Alzheimer's Association published in 2015, only 45 percent of people with Alzheimer's disease are told their diagnosis by their physicians. A much lower percentage (27 percent) are told about having other forms of dementia such as frontotemporal or Lewy body dementia.[1] Fortunately for those of us trying to eliminate dementia stigma and encourage dementia inclusiveness, these famous people had doctors willing to break the news to them.

President Reagan was diagnosed with Alzheimer's disease in 1994, five years after his second term ended. Immediately upon hearing the results of his tests, he requested some writing paper, sat at a small round table in the clinic, and wrote a moving letter to the American people. In it he said, "In opening our hearts, we hope this might promote greater awareness of this condition. Perhaps it will encourage a clearer understanding of the individuals and families who are affected by it."[2] He and his wife, Nancy, then went home to his beloved ranch and asked his assistant to type up his handwritten letter, which ended with this poignant statement: "I now begin the journey that will lead me into the sunset of my life." The journey took 10 years and ended with his death in 2004.[3]

Justice Sandra Day O'Connor was the first woman to serve on the US Supreme Court. She resigned from the court in 2005, saying that she needed to devote her attention to her husband who had been diagnosed with dementia. He died in 2009, and nine years later, at age 88, she received her own dementia diagnosis. Like President Reagan, she chose to go public, saying that she wanted to be open about the changes she was experiencing while she was still able to do that. In her own letter to the American people she recounted her efforts to reinvigorate the teaching of civics and spoke of her gratitude for her opportunities to serve her country.[4]

Country-music singer and songwriter Glen Campbell also made his Alzheimer's disease diagnosis public. Diagnosed in 2011, he embarked on a farewell tour, giving his final show in 2012. His wife supported him in this public effort because she was concerned about people's reactions if he flubbed a line on stage or showed some confusion when performing. In the last concert of the tour, he struggled to sing the words of songs he had performed hundreds of times, but his audience knew about his situation and responded with love and appreciation.

Beloved British author of over 40 fantasy novels, Sir Terry Pratchett chose a different route for informing people about his diagnosis in 2007 at age 59 of a rare form of early-onset Alzheimer's disease (posterior cortical atrophy). He agreed to allow BBC documentary filmmakers to follow him for a year. Pratchett referred to his condition as an "embuggerance" and said that he wanted to "tell everybody" and that he was "not going down without a fight."[5] Toward the end of that year of filming, he struggled to find letters on his keyboard and to read his work aloud. Pratchett, who died in 2015, donated $1 million for Alzheimer's research.

Finally, the sports world was shaken when the woman who had coached more wins than any other college basketball coach announced that at age 59 she, too, had been diagnosed with Alzheimer's disease. Pat Summitt, head coach of the University of Tennessee women's basketball team for 38 years, never had a losing season. Her grit and determination on the basketball court generalized to her response to her diagnosis: "There's not going to be a pity party, and I'll make sure of that."[6] Shortly after her diagnosis, she and her son established the Pat Summitt Foundation to support education about Alzheimer's disease.

These public announcements had their intended effect: people paid attention. A *New York Times* article published a few weeks after Justice O'Connor's announcement described a care-partner support group that met at the Penn Memory Center in Philadelphia. The group's participants all wanted to talk about O'Connor's letter. They said that it made them hopeful that perhaps others might be more understanding of what it was like to care for a person with a stigmatized diagnosis that often left all of them feeling lonely and isolated. They had experienced others withdrawing, treating them with pity, and making them feel shamed and vulnerable.[7] As Pratchett said in an interview included in the BBC documentary, it's important to normalize Alzheimer's disease and other dementias, to bring them out of the shadow of stigma, so that people can talk about them openly.

Apart from these five generally well-known people, many others similarly diagnosed have also stepped up to bear witness to their diagnoses. They have written books, blogs, social-media posts, and insightful comments on websites that serve diagnosed persons and care partners. They have allowed researchers to peer into their lives by participating in interviews and completing surveys. In the United Kingdom, they have also begun to design research studies through the Dementia Enquirers group, a project of the DEEP (Dementia Engagement and Empowerment Project) organization.[8] Their voices are being heard more as worldwide efforts to create dementia-inclusive communities spread.

One could write an entire book about the many topics addressed in writings by people living with dementia—and indeed it has been done.[9] These first-person accounts about life with dementia as diagnosed persons and as care partners cover many topics, but the one most pertinent to life in community concerns their feelings about social connection, in that other people either support or squelch their ability to live with dignity, hope, and meaning.

When Professors Have Dementia

Research shows that the risk of developing dementia increases if a person has no more than a high-school education.[10] People who have earned a bachelor's degree or an advanced degree may have a decreased risk of developing Alzheimer's disease or another dementia. Exposure to higher education and similar cognitive challenges may build "cognitive reserve" by stimulating a more complex web of neural connections in the brain, thus allowing it to compensate, at least initially, for a cognitive impairment.[11] Thus, there may be a delay in developing debilitating symptoms.

Nevertheless, there is also evidence, both from researchers and from first-person accounts, that even people with advanced degrees can develop dementia. And sometimes people with such graduate degrees—especially those who have worked in academia—write books about their experiences, lending their voices to our new narrative.

Cary Henderson, for example, was one of the first professors to write about having dementia. He was 55 years old and not at all ready to stop teaching history at James Madison University when he was diagnosed with younger-onset Alzheimer's disease. With support from his department, he continued to teach part time, but two years later, it was clear to everyone that he could not continue.

Six years after his diagnosis, his wife, Ruth, and their daughter, along with a *Washington Post* photographer, helped Henderson create a remarkable insider account of his daily life over the course of about 10 months. Using a cassette tape recorder, he spoke about what gave him joy and what caused him to despair. He called the book *Partial View* because, he believed, "The best thing to do about this is just not worry about it. Be happy with the partial view or whatever else is partial, everything is partial."[12] By the time the book was published, his view of the world had narrowed considerably. As Ruth recounted in her introduction to the book, his family had to make the difficult decision that he needed to live in a nursing home when his condition became severe. In the poignant words of the Global Deterioration Scale, an early staging model of Alzheimer's disease, his "brain [appeared] to no longer be able to tell the body what to do."[13] Nevertheless, Ruth observed what she described as a "tiny spark" remaining in him, because when she told him the book would be published, his eyes filled with tears that she interpreted as tears of joy.

Henderson was acutely aware of dementia stigma. Speaking into the tape recorder, he said:

> I would love to see some people with Alzheimer's not trying to stay in the shadows all the time, but to say, damn it, we're people too. And we want to be talked to and respected as if we were honest-to-God real people.[14]

Frustrations about his ability to communicate appear frequently in Henderson's descriptions of life with dementia. He talked about how his thinking had slowed and his words got tangled, so that he had trouble participating in conversations. This inability to communicate made him aware of how socially isolated he had become. For example, he said:

> And another really crazy thing about Alzheimer's, nobody really wants to talk to you any longer. They're maybe afraid of us. I don't know if that's the trouble or not, I assume it is, but we can assure everybody that we know Alzheimer's is not catching.[15]

This theme of social isolation continued in his reflections, including this one:

> I think one of the worst things about Alzheimer's is you're so alone with it. Nobody around you really knows what's going on. And half the time, most of the time, we don't know what's going on ourselves. I would like some exchange of views, exchange of experiences, and I think for me at least, this is a very important part of life.[16]

For several years after his diagnosis, Cary and Ruth Henderson made regular 400-mile round trips so he could participate in a research study at Duke University. In the introduction to his book, Ruth described how his years in the study added meaning to his life and connected him with a community of researchers who treated them like friends. The thought of helping others through his participation in their research gave him hope, and he relished the dignity conferred on him by the team at Duke. He felt like a fully accepted citizen of this research community. This is what he said about his research participation:

I've thoroughly enjoyed being a guinea pig… They bring me back to Durham almost all the time—whenever they need whatever it is, some of my blood or something else, and it's kind of fun. I feel like I'm doing something not only interesting but I think something that's needed… It's something that I can do that not everybody can do, and it makes me feel very good about this. It makes me feel like I'm not going to just rot in my old age, helpless and stupid.[17]

Richard Taylor, another former professor, knew what it was like to feel helpless and stupid. As I mentioned in Chapter 2, Richard's doctor told him that he had "dementia, probably of the Alzheimer's type." When Taylor, a clinical psychologist and psychology professor, received that diagnosis at age 58 in 2002 he experienced considerable emotional trauma. He said that he hid from the rest of the world, had anxiety and depression, and felt no purpose in his life, especially after he had to resign from his teaching position and give up his practice. Fortunately, he decided that hiding in an imaginary closet was the wrong approach. What he most needed was to retain a sense of normality, as well as affirmation of his social citizenship—that is, affirmation of his right to be valued as a contributing member of society who can be of service to others. He reoriented himself by writing the 82 essays that eventually became his book *Alzheimer's from the Inside Out*.

Taylor said that writing became his "therapy without a co-pay."[18] A major turning point happened when he showed some of his essays to a friend who also had early-onset Alzheimer's disease. The friend appreciated what he wrote and recommended his writings to others. This friend's response nurtured Taylor's passion for encouraging people with dementia to support one another by creating social networks in neighborhoods through what he called "hello dinners." This was his way of creating a dementia-inclusive and friendly community serving not only people having dementia but also neighbors, who he thought should get to know people living with the condition.

In addition to writing the essays for his book, Taylor created a website, recorded YouTube lectures, wrote an e-newsletter, produced two DVDs, and traveled all over the world speaking at meetings of organizations dedicated to making it possible for persons with dementia to live as well as possible. He wanted these fellow travelers to feel better about themselves and to uphold their identities as whole persons, because he knew all too well that others often viewed them only in terms of what was missing.

Taylor had strong opinions about advocacy and activism, a topic I will address in the next chapter. Though he intentionally encouraged community connections in a variety of ways, the strain of social isolation was another theme running through his work. Like Henderson, he noted that people seemed not to want to talk with him once they knew his diagnosis. He expressed it like this:

> I have become keenly aware of a patterned response from some individuals as soon as they find out I have Alzheimer's disease. They switch their eye contact and attention to whomever I am with. It is as if knowledge of the disease immediately cloaks me in invisibility.[19]

Many people treated Taylor as if he were invisible, turning to address his wife or adult children when they found out he had Alzheimer's. He understood that their behavior betrayed their ignorance of how to communicate with him. He urged people to greet a person with dementia by saying "hello." He understood that his memory and word-finding problems made communicating with him difficult, but he wanted people to try to reach him by looking him in the eyes and being patient listeners.

Taylor said that treating another person as if he or she is invisible is a way of turning that person into an "It" (with a capital "I")—an object to be used and controlled. The work of theologian and philosopher Martin Buber inspired Taylor to make these observations. Buber distinguished between objectifying another person as an "It" and honoring that person as a whole person, a "Thou."[20] Taylor was acutely aware of how his dementia symptoms affected his relationships with the people he loved. He said that sometimes they treated him as an "It" but that sometimes he treated them as "Its." Here is how Taylor expressed his feelings about the changes he knew were happening in himself and thus in his relationships:

> I am no longer who I formerly was. I am no longer like everyone, but there is still a good deal of me left. Am I half empty or half full?

What difference does it make in terms of being a full and equal member of the family? It's tough for everyone!

My heart aches and I want to shout: "I'm a different Thou, not a quarter It and three quarters Thou."[21]

Cary Henderson and Richard Taylor wanted others to treat them with dignity. While meaning for Henderson came from his participation in the research studies at Duke University, Taylor derived meaning from the enormous web of relationships developed after his diagnosis through his writing and speaking. Both understood the benefits for themselves and their care partners of dementia inclusivity.

Three Strong Women

Like Richard Taylor, Helga Rohra (from Germany) and Christine Bryden and Kate Swaffer (both from Australia) have been tireless advocates for social change in attitudes and public policies that affect the lives of people having dementia. They interacted with one another by attending the same conferences and working with organizations such as Alzheimer's Disease International. In fact, Swaffer has said that it was Taylor's writings that inspired her to come out with her diagnosis and to become actively engaged in "living beyond the diagnosis of dementia."[22] I will describe their activism and advocacy efforts in the next chapter, but for now, I want to include them here because they, too, have written books about living with dementia.

Similar to Henderson and Taylor, Rohra, Bryden, and Swaffer were diagnosed in their late 40s to early 50s. All three women have been actively involved in international organizations and have campaigned for inclusion of persons having dementia in these organizations. They want to be fully accepted as participants, and they refuse to be treated as some kind of sideshow apart from the "real" work of the conference done by researchers and politicians.[23] Also, they speak for persons diagnosed with some type of dementia before age 65—the younger-onset people having dementia with Lewy bodies (Rohra), frontotemporal dementia (Bryden), and Alzheimer's dementia (Swaffer).

Helga Rohra's book speaks directly to the situation encountered by people whose dementia diagnosis comes before age 65.[24] Hers came at age 50, a time when she was actively involved in her professional life as a teacher, linguist, and translator in Germany. In addition to the financial impact of not being able to work as much, the diagnosis presented a number of challenges to her social identity. For example, she said that she did not feel elderly even though most people associate dementia with older adults. Also, Rohra writes that she is twice divorced and raising her son who has Asperger's syndrome. She notes that many programs for persons living with dementia assume that the person can call upon close family connections for support—something she cannot do.

Proudly independent, Rohra admits that it is hard for her to ask others for help. This is a challenging balancing act, because while she advises against overprotecting people having dementia, she also recognizes that respectful assistance is sometimes necessary. She embraces the essential human need for meaningful social relationships, stating in her book that it has always mattered to her to be in touch with people. In recent years she has developed many significant relationships internationally through her efforts in founding the European Working Group of People with Dementia.[25]

Australian Christine Bryden has written four books and a number of journal articles.[26] Like Rohra, she has traveled worldwide giving lectures on her life with dementia, insisting that she wants to be treated with respect and empathy. Many of these lectures can be found on YouTube. Also like Rohra, Bryden speaks forcefully about what she calls the "toxic lie of dementia"—the assumption that people having dementia have completely lost their minds, are capable of nothing, and exist only as empty shells.

Although Rohra stated in her book that she is not a regular churchgoer, she did say that she finds strength through her belief in God, prayer, and meditation. Bryden speaks more directly about her faith, saying that she finds comfort in her Christian beliefs and the possibility for spiritual growth and healing because of, not in spite of, her dementia. Writing in a journal article she coauthored with her spiritual director, Elizabeth MacKinlay, Bryden talked about how dementia stigma limited others' views of her ability to flourish spiritually:

This stigma leads to restrictions on our ability to develop our spirituality. It threatens our spiritual identity. It is assumed that the limits due to our failing cognition place us beyond reach of normal spiritual practices, of communion with God and with others.[27]

To combat the toxic lie, she wants people to focus on her soul and not her mind, the latter of which, she says, produces "my odd behavior, my lack of social graces, my lack of resources to offer in friendship."[28]

Bryden, a biochemist who, after her diagnosis at age 46, completed a postgraduate diploma in pastoral care and counseling, is acutely aware of how others view her. She has lived with her condition for over 20 years, a fact that has forced her to endure many instances of the insulting comments experienced by Taylor, Rohra, Swaffer, and others. Often, for example, people doubt their diagnoses and say, "You don't look like you have dementia."

Another Australian who does not look like she has dementia, and who would be insulted by anyone who said that, is Kate Swaffer. Diagnosed at age 49, she is widely known for her description of what she and many others experience when given the dementia diagnosis: Prescribed Disengagement™. She trademarked that phrase and uses it often in her writing and public speaking.[29] It resulted from her doctor telling her to stop working and studying; he gave her a pathway not for living but for dying. Swaffer also believes that instead of focusing solely on medications, physicians should pay attention to exercise, diet, and activities of community engagement, such as blogging, advocacy, and volunteering. Ten years after she trademarked Prescribed Disengagement, Swaffer wrote in a blog post that she hears from others that the advice to give up and prepare to die is still being given.

Since her diagnosis, Swaffer has formed many new relationships with others like her who want to advocate for themselves. She is one of the cofounders of Dementia Alliance International (DAI), a group of people with dementia who declared that they no longer wanted others to speak for them.[30] Inspired by Richard Taylor's plea for people to say "hello" to one another, DAI has produced a series of short "Hello" videos by people introducing themselves and talking about what it is like for them to live with dementia—or, as Swaffer would say, to live *beyond* dementia.[31]

Swaffer has strong opinions about how people having dementia are treated. For example, she is tired of hearing that they are a burden and need to be locked up. She resists the stigmatizing language often used when people talk about those with dementia, even objecting when the word "memory" (as in "memory loss") is used in the title of so many programs, because memory is not always the primary problem for people with certain types of dementia.

Today, thanks to the courageous leadership of Rohra, Bryden, Swaffer, and many others, people with dementia are speaking up and speaking out about how they want to be treated. Each has a unique story to tell, though with similar themes. For example, in a DAI blog post, American writer, artist, and filmmaker Minna Packer describes why she believes that her PTSD from growing up as the child of Holocaust survivors made her Alzheimer's symptoms worse.[32] Packer has experienced people she thought were friends withdrawing from her and failing to answer her emails and phone calls, an experience shared by others described in this chapter.

Who's Missing?

Books and blogs by persons living with some type of dementia have proliferated in recent years. Most are by relatively young individuals like many of the people introduced in this chapter. While celebrating the worldwide impact of the persons named here, we need to ask, Whose voices are not being heard? In her most recent book, Kate Swaffer offers this list: those who are LGBTIQ, aboriginal, homeless, intellectually disabled, indigenous, culturally and linguistically diverse (CALD),[33] and living alone.

I would add another large and growing group of persons: those whose dementia has progressed to the point that relocation to some type of care community has become necessary. This is one of the greatest fears of persons having dementia, a fear often expressed by Cary Henderson in his tape-recorded musings about his life with dementia. Similarly, in a 2012 lecture to the Aged Care Quality and Safety Commission in Australia, Christine Bryden described her dread of being placed in a "dementia prison."[34] She talked about her visits to many memory-care residences where she observed how people with dementia were treated as objects to be "physically cared for by the harassed and over-worked staff." How can we hear the voices of these people living with dementia, given the fact that their wider communities often behave as if their residences are invisible? Although community members may pass these residences daily, unless they work there, or a loved one lives there, they probably know little about the people for whom this is home.

At the present time, the best ways I know to learn about how people feel about living in a long-term-care community are to talk with them or to read reports of research studies using qualitative methods. "Qualitative" usually means that the investigators have interviewed people and have then subjected the interview transcriptions to a rigorous analysis. A good example comes from the work of Linda Clare and her colleagues (introduced in Chapter 2). They began one of their papers with this statement: "The subjective psychological experience of people with moderate to severe dementia living in residential care is insufficiently understood."[35]

The researchers conducted multiple unstructured, recorded conversations with 81 British people living in 10 different residential care homes. This process produced 304 conversations analyzed for their common themes. Consistent with the analytic approach they employed, Clare and her colleagues identified four themes using the words of those they interviewed: "Nothing's right now," "I'm all right; I'll manage," "I am still somebody," and "It drives me mad." Here are some quotes from residents included in the paper:

> "I'm so lonely here. I don't know what's the matter with me, and what's the matter...why people don't talk to me much. I feel to be an outsider."[36]

> "You just wish you didn't have to come in here... I just wish my family would show up now and again."[37]

> "I feel I'm not attached to me family."[38]

> "Don't lose me, will you? Please don't lose me."[39]

> "I'm an old woman and nobody wants me. I mean, that's the case, nobody does. If I was wanted by anybody, I'd go, and I could be quite useful. But nobody knows that I want a job."[40]

These quotes and many others appearing in their paper led Clare and her research team to conclude this: "The experience of living with dementia in residential care was fundamentally one of experiencing difficult and distressing emotions relating to loss, isolation, uncertainty, fear, and a sense of worthlessness."[41] This statement echoes the observations of Dr. Bill Thomas, founder of The Eden Alternative, an organization focused on changing the culture of care through its vision of eliminating the loneliness, helplessness, and boredom experienced by too many elders, especially those having dementia.[42]

Loneliness. Helplessness. Boredom. This is what Christine Bryden observed when she visited the memory-care residences in Australia. These feelings gnaw at the innermost core of people's being. In a 2012 lecture, which is on YouTube,[43] she begged her audience of policy makers and care providers to focus on the emotional and spiritual needs of residents, to see them as "people, not disease burdens." Bryden clearly saw that care communities need to find creative ways to help people with dementia develop meaningful connections with other people, feel as if they still have something meaningful to give to others, and engage in meaningful activities.

The Lonely Care Partner

In 2008, when I was on sabbatical and interviewing people living with dementia (including care partners) about their friendship networks, I visited many private homes in northeast Wisconsin. I vividly recall sitting at a kitchen table in a farmhouse and talking with a middle-aged woman about her loneliness as a care partner. She was caring for her father who had Alzheimer's dementia, helping her husband on the farm, and raising four energetic children. While their pet parrot squawked in the background, this woman told me, "People just don't come around here much anymore. They don't know what to say." Despite her days being fully occupied with caring for her family and doing the work of a farmer, this woman felt an inner emptiness and a disconnection from the community she had grown up in.

In this chapter we have heard from persons living with a dementia about their feelings of being excluded and ignored by others. Sometimes those others are medical professionals. For example, Lucy Whitman, editor of a collection of first-person accounts of experiences of caring for loved ones with dementia, told her own story of exclusion when her mother was admitted to the hospital because of "spells" resulting from urinary tract infections and an earlier fall. Her mother was hospitalized for five weeks, and during that time her mental acuity declined precipitously. However, no doctor, nurse, or social worker ever acknowledged to Whitman or her sister what was happening. This is how Whitman described this harrowing time:

> Not one person acknowledged that our mother had suddenly plunged into an advanced state of dementia; not one person sat us down and talked about what this might mean for our mother and for the rest of the family.

> ...It did not seem to occur to them that a sudden steep deterioration in mental function should be taken just as seriously as any marked physical change. Even if there was nothing they could do about it, they should have been prepared to talk to us about what was going on.

When her mother was finally being released from the hospital, Whitman attempted to get information from a social worker about how to care for her mother. This is what happened:

> I then received another call from the social worker, telling me in an exasperated way that she had not been able to get any sense out of my mother, to find out what her needs were, because "she's completely demented!" Throughout her long stay in hospital, the word dementia had never once been uttered by the nurses or doctors, even in response to all the concerns we had expressed. For it to be mentioned in this brutally casual way was like being stabbed in the heart.[44]

Dementia care partners writing in articles, books, blogs, and social-media posts share many stories about feeling socially excluded and denied the dignity of being treated respectfully. In perusing the caregiving research literature and the growing number of first-person accounts of the stresses and frequent social isolation experienced by those caring for someone with dementia, I wondered again about whose voices were missing. In other words, Swaffer's list of the missing applies to care partners as well as to persons having dementia.[45]

Two very different experiences introduced me to persons representing groups on Swaffer's list. One took place in Oslo, Norway, and the other happened as I sat in front of my computer in Appleton, Wisconsin.

In Oslo, in 2008, I was attending a meeting of Alzheimer Europe and had the good fortune to be assigned to stand with my poster next to a man named Roger Newman, who also had prepared a poster. Newman, a caregiver for his partner, David, had designed this poster to highlight the fact that the Alzheimer's Society of the UK had supported him in founding an LGBT carers' group. He and I chatted at length and later corresponded through email. Newman felt that his poster was necessary because the literature he had received from the Alzheimer's Society appeared to exclude the LGBT community. As he notes in his personal account in Lucy Whitman's book, the Alzheimer's Society had seemed to support the erroneous belief that "the disease only affected married couples or those with supportive families. The focus seemed to be on heroic husbands or wives, married for scores of years, or devoted sons and daughters."[46]

Even though Newman's partner was diagnosed at a young age, at 52, he aged visibly as his dementia progressed, leading some to assume that he was Newman's father. This forced them to tell others that they were partners, a relationship that made some people uncomfortable.

Their own discomfort increased dramatically when David had to relocate to a residential home. They missed the gay world they had created over many years together. In a chapter included in Whitman's book, Newman wrote: "We had built a wall around our relationship that made us feel that it was easy being a gay couple... The onset of David's dementia, however, turned everything upside down."[47] For Newman, the loneliness of dementia caregiving was intensified by the social attitudes about homosexuality that he and David had encountered throughout their lives. When people commented that attitudes about LGBT persons had changed, he thought:

> They do not realize that older gay men and lesbians bring with us, to this task of caring, a significant amount of baggage from a previous age. The men remember all too clearly being "illegal" and being

victims of police harassment. The women remember a society where people hardly believed that lesbians actually existed.[48]

Newman's experience made me wonder if other groups of people have voices that are seldom heard in first-person writings about having dementia or being a care partner. As I pondered this, I scrolled through the website of a subgroup of the organization UsAgainstAlzheimer's.[49] On the page for African Americans Against Alzheimer's, I learned about a book Loretta Veney wrote about caring for her mother, Doris.

Reflecting findings from research on African Americans caring for family members with dementia, Veney tells the story of a tightly knit family working hard to give the best possible care to her mother. Like Roger Newman and David, Veney and Doris had to cope not only with dementia symptoms but also with negative social attitudes and dementia fear. For example, she wrote about the patience and tolerance she had to develop when people stared at her mother and commented "under their breaths about how often she repeated herself."[50] People even jokingly told Veney that they would kill themselves if their mother repeated things all the time.

Eventually it was no longer safe for her mother to live alone, so Veney had to move quickly to find a place for her mother to live safely and happily. Fortunately, there was space available at a group home called Mamie's Loving Care. With only six residents, Ms. Mamie's place felt like an actual home. Veney's first visit came during lunchtime when all the residents were sitting at the dining-room table. What struck Veney about this scene was the camaraderie she observed:

> Even though they all couldn't recall each other's names, they were interacting and engaged in friendly small talk. Those expressions of communal fellowship are what I consider the simple pleasures of life. Two of the residents were looking out of the windows commenting to each other on how beautiful a day it was. To observe two 95-year-olds chatting so amiably was thrilling for me.[51]

In this small, intimate, caring community of African American elders, Veney felt confident that her mother would not suffer from the three plagues of elder care identified by The Eden Alternative: loneliness, helplessness, and boredom.

What Have They Taught Us?

We have come a long way from the famous people mentioned at the beginning of this chapter. We have heard from some professors with dementia and other men and women with international reputations for advocacy and activism on behalf of persons having dementia. How many other stories are waiting to be told by people with the diagnosis, or by people caring for someone with a dementia? Whose voices are still not being heard? What do they have to teach us?

One common theme in stories told both by people living with dementia and by care partners points to the importance of caring, supportive, inclusive communities. In these communities, people having dementia can live with dignity, hope, and meaning.

Dignity is relational; it is grounded in interpersonal interactions. We confer dignity upon one another in our relationships, but other people can also subvert our dignity through the ways they relate to us. Roger Newman experienced that as he tried to navigate care systems seeking a place for David to live. Loretta Veney experienced assaults on her mother's dignity when people whispered behind her back and sometimes stated to her face that her mother was repeating herself. Cary Henderson and Richard Taylor longed for others to treat them with dignity, and Helga Rohra, Christine Bryden, and Kate Swaffer continue to remind their audiences that they are, as Bryden puts it, "people, not disease burdens."

Hope is also relational. The current popular definition of hope about dementia is hope for a cure. Of course, everyone in what some refer to as "dementia world"—persons with the symptoms and diagnoses, care partners, and professionals of various types working in this field—hopes that one day no one will have any type of dementia. However, that hope is usually centered on biomedical goals to cure people of the brain changes associated with the dementias. What the voices heard here seem to be saying is that their hope is for acceptance and inclusion, and for support for lives that are meaningful regardless of where they happen to be in the progression of dementia. Because this type of hope is not nearly as well publicized as the hope for a cure, many of these individuals have discovered that they need to become advocates and activists in order to change attitudes about dementia and ensure that the human rights of people living with dementia are honored.

Endnotes

1   Contrast this finding with the study's report of a disclosure rate of over 90 percent for various cancers: Alzheimer's Association. (2015). *2015 Alzheimer's disease facts and figures*. Chicago, IL: Alzheimer's Association. Accessed on 7/13/19 at www.alz.org/media/documents/2015factsandfigures.pdf

2   The story about President and Mrs. Reagan receiving the diagnosis appears in a new biography by Bob Spitz: Spitz, B. (2018). *Reagan: An American journey*. New York, NY: Penguin Press.

   President Reagan's letter can be found at www.reaganlibrary.gov/sreference/reagan-s-letter-announcing-his-alzheimer-s-diagnosis

3   Books about Ronald Reagan fill library shelves, but one in particular focuses on his life after he left the White House: Shirley, C. (2015). *Last act: The final years and emerging legacy of Ronald Reagan*. Nashville, TN: Nelson Books.

4   Justice O'Connor's letter can be found at https://int.nyt.com/data/documenthelper/403-sandra-day-oconnor-letter-dementia/d88af3d08c563a566fc4/optimized/full.pdf#page=1

5   Part one of the BBC documentary *Living with Alzheimer's* appears at www.youtube.com/watch?v=KmejLjxFmCQ

   Part two appears at www.youtube.com/watch?v=tTgqocgY5Ww

6   Gregory, S. (2011, August 11). Pat Summitt's toughest opponent yet: Early onset dementia. *TIME*. Accessed on 7/17/19 at http://newsfeed.time.com/2011/08/24/pat-summitts-toughest-opponent-yet-early-onset-dementia

7   Span, P. (2018, November 12). The increasingly public face of dementia. *New York Times*, p. D6.

8   See www.dementiavoices.org.uk/dementia-enquirers for more information about this group.

9   Martina Zimmerman's goal was to consider all books published by people with dementia and care partners over a 30-year period. However, because there are many more books by care partners than by those with dementia, she had to be selective about the ones she analyzed. She showed how greater worldwide awareness of dementia coincided with an increase in the number of these works and how, during this period, a person-centered focus became more dominant. Grounded in narrative theory, her work reflects critical scholarship of illness narratives: Zimmerman, M. (2017). *The poetics and politics of Alzheimer's disease life-writing*. Cham, Switzerland: Palgrave Macmillan.

   See also a chapter titled "Autobiographies by people with dementia" in Anne Basting's book: Basting, A. (2009). *Forget memory: Creating better lives for people with dementia*. Baltimore, MD: Johns Hopkins University Press.

10 Hussenoeder, F. S., & Riedel-Heller, S. G. (2018). Primary prevention of dementia: From modifiable risk factors to a public brain health agenda? *Social Psychiatry and Psychiatric Epidemiology, 53*, 1289–1301.

11 Leggett, A., Clarke, P., Zivin, K., McCammon, R. J., Elliott, M. R., & Langa, K. M. (2019). Recent improvements in cognitive functioning among older US adults: How much does increasing educational attainment explain? *Journals of Gerontology: Social Sciences, 74*, 536–545.

12 Cary Henderson received the Alzheimer's diagnosis in an unusual way. He had a brain shunt inserted for what doctors thought was normal pressure hydrocephalus (it wasn't). His wife, having noticed some changes in his thinking, asked if Alzheimer's might be a possibility. The neurosurgeon removed a small bit of tissue, and this is how he became one of the first living people to have Alzheimer's disease diagnosed based on the presence of neurofibrillary tangles and plaques. Ordinarily, that conclusion comes from autopsy, although there are also cases in the literature—most famously from the nuns' study—where autopsied brains have shown the characteristic signs of Alzheimer's dementia but the individuals had developed no discernible symptoms. Henderson, C. S. (1998). *Partial view: An Alzheimer's journal.* Dallas, TX: Southern Methodist University, epigraph.

    Snowdon, D. (2001). *Aging with grace: What the Nun Study teaches us about leading longer, healthier, and more meaningful lives.* New York, NY: Bantam Books.

13 Reisberg, B., Ferris, S. H., DeLeon, M. J., & Crook, T. (1982). The Global Deterioration Scale for assessment of primary degenerative dementia. *American Journal of Psychiatry, 139*, 1136–1139. (p. 1138)

14 Henderson, p. 7.

15 Henderson, p. 18.

16 Henderson, p. 55.

17 Henderson, p. 60 and p. 63.

18 Taylor, R. (2007). *Alzheimer's from the inside out.* Baltimore, MD: Health Professions Press. (p. xvii)

19 Taylor, p. 152.

20 Buber's work, especially his writing about I/Thou relationships, was a major influence on Tom Kitwood as he developed his ideas about the personhood of people having dementia: Buber, M. (1970). *I and Thou* (W. Kaufman, Trans.). New York, NY: Charles Scribner's Sons.

21 Taylor, p. 151.

22 Swaffer, K. (2016). *What the hell happened to my brain? Living beyond dementia.* Philadelphia, PA: Jessica Kingsley Publishers. (p. 29)

23 In her book *Forget memory*, Anne Basting describes meeting Richard Taylor at a conference. She notes the "sideshow" problem at some meetings, but Taylor was definitely not a sideshow. Basting recognized that of all the conference's speakers, he had the most expertise about dementia because he lived with it 24/7.

24 Rohra, H. (2016). *Dementia activist: Fighting for our rights.* London, UK: Jessica Kingsley Publishers.

25 In 2012, my husband, John, and I had the pleasure of meeting Helga Rohra on a bus in Vienna, Austria. We were going with a group of attendees at the Alzheimer Europe conference to the annual gala, a fancy and fun event held that year in an ancient underground restaurant that featured a collection of antique hats. The European Working Group ensures that people with dementia have meaningful roles participating in Alzheimer Europe conferences: www.alzheimer-europe.org/Alzheimer-Europe/Who-we-are/European-Working-Group-of-People-with-Dementia/(language)/eng-GB

26 Bryden's books all have compelling titles:

Bryden, C. (2005). *Dancing with dementia: My story of living positively with dementia*. London, UK: Jessica Kingsley Publishers.

Bryden, C. (2012). *Who will I be when I die?* London, UK: Jessica Kingsley Publishers.

Bryden, C. (2015). *Nothing about us without us: 20 years of dementia advocacy*. London, UK: Jessica Kingsley Publishers.

Bryden, C. (2015). *Before I forget: How I survived younger-onset dementia*. London, UK: e-Penguin.

27 Bryden, C., & MacKinlay, E. (2002). Dementia—A spiritual journey towards the divine: A personal view of dementia. In E. MacKinlay (Ed.), *Mental health and spirituality in later life* (pp. 69–75). Binghamton, NY: Haworth Pastoral Press. (p. 71)

28 Bryden & MacKinlay, p. 73.

29 Swaffer, K. (2016). *What the hell happened to my brain? Living beyond dementia*. Philadelphia, PA: Jessica Kingsley Publishers.

30 Dementia Alliance International (www.dementiaallianceinternational.org), in association with Alzheimer's Disease International, brings people together from throughout the world to advocate for persons having dementia. They describe themselves as the "global voice of dementia" and emphasize the human rights of persons with dementia. They aim to demonstrate how to "live beyond the diagnosis of dementia."

31 www.dementiaallianceinternational.org/services/hello-our-voices-matter

32 Minna Packer describes her PTSD symptoms in a DAI online article: www.dementiaallianceinternational.org/minnas-story-dementia-and-ptsd

33 This category—CALD—is used in Australia to describe persons called "racially and ethnically diverse" in the US. It is viewed as preferable since race and ethnicity are socially constructed terms with no inherent biological basis.

34 Aged Care Quality and Safety Commission. (2013). *Christine Bryden: Dreading being put in dementia prison*. Accessed on 9/30/19 at www.youtube.com/watch?v=V1GDQ0vhLTY

35 Clare, L., Rowlands, J., Bruce, E., Surr, C., & Downs, M. (2008). The experience of living with dementia in residential care: An interpretive phenomenological analysis. *The Gerontologist, 48*, 711–720. (p. 711)

36 Clare et al., p. 715.

37 Clare et al., p. 715.

38 Clare et al., p. 715.

39 Clare et al., p. 716.

40 Clare et al., p. 716.

41 Clare et al., p. 711.

42 Thomas, W. H. (1996). *Life worth living: How someone you love can still enjoy life in a nursing home—The Eden Alternative in action*. Acton, MA: VanderWyk & Burnham.

See also the website for The Eden Alternative and the statements about its mission, vision, values, and principles: www.edenalt.org/about-the-eden-alternative/mission-vision-values

43 www.youtube.com/watch?v=V1GDQ0vhLTY&t=15s

44 Whitman, L. (2010). On the contrary. In L. Whitman (Ed.), *Telling tales about dementia: Experiences of caring* (pp. 93–102). Philadelphia, PA: Jessica Kingsley Publishers. (pp. 97–98)

45 Helga Rohra's group, the European Working Group of People with Dementia, along with researchers working with Alzheimer Europe, produced a detailed, scholarly report called *The Development of Intercultural Care and Support for People with Dementia from Minority Ethnic Groups*. A full-text version is available online (www.researchgate.net/publication/331438946); a hard copy can be ordered from Alzheimer Europe.

46 Newman, R. (2010). Surely the world has changed? In L. Whitman (Ed.), *Telling tales about dementia: Experiences of caring* (pp. 145–151). Philadelphia, PA: Jessica Kingsley Publishers. (p. 150)

47 Newman, p. 146.

48 Newman, p. 150.

49 www.usagainstalzheimers.org/about

50 Veney, L. A. W. (2012). *Being my mom's mom: A journey through dementia from a daughter's perspective.* West Conshohocken, PA: Infinity Publishing. (p. 102)

51 Veney, pp. 89–90.

Chapter 5

Dementia Advocacy and Activism

Richard Taylor concluded his book *Alzheimer's from the Inside Out* about his experiences living with dementia with these exclamations: *Act Up! Ring Out! SPEAK UP and OUT!*[1] He named a number of pressing concerns in his last, brief entry, the first being how hard it is for people having dementia to obtain disability insurance. It was particularly challenging in his state of Texas. Taylor's activism and advocacy may have contributed to the fact that, three years after the publication of his book in 2007, the Social Security Administration included younger/early-onset Alzheimer's disease in its CAL (Compassionate Allowances) Initiative. This means that persons younger than 65 who are diagnosed with Alzheimer's disease or one of eight other types of dementia qualify for expedited access to Social Security Disability Insurance (SSDI).

Taylor also offered a poignant description of what happens to people with more advanced dementia who require long-term care and must pay for it themselves. It comes as a shock to many Americans that Medicare does not cover this type of long-term care. If you are very wealthy, you can afford to hire 24/7 in-home care or you can pay for residential care. If you are poor, the Medicaid program will cover some of your costs. However, if you are neither rich nor poor you will need to spend down your assets so that you become poor, and then you may qualify for Medicaid benefits. Taylor observed this:

> …after we have lost our sense of self, our sense of dignity, we fall into a shaky and shrinking Medicaid system that no one wants to

fund but everyone wants to keep as a "safety net" for their parents, and perhaps for themselves. We slip from one end of the long-term care facility with the fresh flowers and private rooms to the bare Medicaid wards in distant wings of the facility.[2]

Taylor was not exaggerating. I have visited a number of nursing homes that have renovated areas for rehabilitation (covered by Medicare because it is considered short term, leading to measurable improvement) and feature carpeting, tasteful lighting, and new furniture. Turn the corner, however, to enter the area where people on Medicaid live, and you walk on linoleum past medicine carts, mechanical lifts, and other equipment lining the halls.

Taylor borrowed his cry of "Act Up!" from the AIDS movement. He said that high levels of funding for AIDS research were not reached because people stayed home and worked in their gardens. He did acknowledge, however, that while many people with AIDS are activists, some may be too ill to participate in rallies and marches; they rely on their friends to join the cause. These friends, said Taylor, "mobilized individuals with an interest in their cause and made acting as an advocate an expected part of dealing with the disease."[3] In the early stages of dementia, people can follow Taylor's advice to write letters, send emails, and speak out in community gatherings, but when such work becomes no longer possible, friends need to step up and become involved in advocacy and activism.

I signed up to receive Taylor's e-newsletter late in 2010. These newsletters were always full of his pithy remarks about life in "dementia world," descriptions of his international travels to raise awareness of what it is like to live with dementia, and his frequent strong objections to policy decisions by the Alzheimer's Association. Then, in 2013, he informed his readers that he was being treated for esophageal cancer.

Taylor died in June 2015, and in August his son posted the newsletter Taylor had begun writing before his death. His son wrote an introductory paragraph, ending it by saying, "The first question I am continually asked is, Who will take Richard's place in this fight? My personal wish is not for any one person to replace him. I would wish to see hundreds, if not thousands, that take his place and all STAND UP AND SPEAK OUT!"[4]

In that newsletter, Taylor had reflected on the growing numbers of people around the world living with some type of dementia and argued that all the money raised to find a cure has not yielded much that helps people living with the condition today. On the other hand, he said, what we do have are communities—communities where people living with dementia could benefit from money invested in psychosocial research to improve their life quality now and to improve the life quality of their care partners. This was a strong theme throughout his post-diagnostic work. In *Alzheimer's from the Inside Out*, he expressed his plea like this:

> At least for a while, there isn't much that can be done about what is happening with the chemistry between my ears, so why not spend time working on what is happening to the chemistry between my spouse and me? Between mothers and daughters? Within families? Among friends?[5]

These questions remain unanswered by most of the multimillion-dollar research studies on Alzheimer's disease and other types of dementia. But Taylor did not want biomedical research on dementia causes and cures to cease. Rather, he wanted more attention to be paid to improving the lives of people currently living with dementia, and he urged that more funding be directed toward research and programs supporting this goal.

Advocacy vs. Activism

Was Richard Taylor an advocate, an activist, or both? I think the answer is "both," but you can quickly slide down a Google rabbit hole by searching for how the terms are different. Long before the internet, when I was in graduate school, I had a professor who talked about people who "bore from within" and those who "hammer from without." Usually the latter is associated with activism, a term that has acquired a negative connotation in some quarters by being associated with protests, some of which get out of control.

Both advocacy and activism involve some kind of action, and often the terms are used interchangeably. Examples of activities that reflect both advocacy and activism include letter writing to policy makers, participating in organized advocacy days for visiting legislators, and walking for a cause and raising money for it. Sometimes people who identify as activists deride people for "just" being advocates, saying that they lack will and courage to really stand up for their cause. However, I find that attitude unhelpful, because both the quiet advocacy of writing letters and the noisy energy of protest marches can stimulate change. The common theme for both advocacy and activism is that people who care about a cause are willing to speak up and out, just as Richard Taylor said. Yes, sometimes that involves some loud hammering from without, but change can also come from quiet and persistent boring from within when people work for change within governments, businesses, nonprofits, faith communities, and other organizations that have some relationship with people living with dementia.

Helga, Christine, and Kate SPEAK UP and OUT!

As I suggested earlier, there is much to learn from the advocacy and activism of Helga Rohra, Christine Bryden, and Kate Swaffer. Diagnosed at a young age and living with different types of dementia, these three women have been speaking up and out for several years at conferences and in their books, journal articles, and blog posts. German activist Rohra even titled her 2011 book in English *Dementia Activist: Fighting for Our Rights*.[6] In it she argues that society is not willing to consider people's competencies when they are diagnosed with a dementia. She is particularly concerned about those like her who receive the diagnosis while still working. She observes that many dementia advocacy groups appear to focus on persons more elderly than she is, leaving her feeling as if her need to experience meaning and purpose through work is not recognized or valued. She also advocates for more resources and support for middle-aged people with dementia who live alone.

As an activist, Rohra started the European Working Group of People with Dementia (EWGPWD) in 2012, five years after her diagnosis with Lewy body disease. This group operates independently of Alzheimer Europe, though as EWGPWD board chair, Rohra also served on the board of Alzheimer Europe until 2018. She has traveled widely and does not hesitate to call out large and small irritations encountered in airports, hotels, and conference centers. Although she firmly states that she and her colleagues with dementia should not be overprotected, she was also instrumental in urging Alzheimer Europe to set aside quiet rooms at its conferences for attendees with dementia. She refuses to be patronized, she objects when people treat her and others like her as helpless children, and she reminds the world that people living with dementia still want to have fun and enjoy leisure activities.

Similarly, Christine Bryden of Australia adopted the disability rights slogan mentioned earlier when she titled one of her books *Nothing About Us Without Us: 20 Years of Dementia Advocacy*.[7] A main concern she has shared in her writing and speaking has been the way nursing homes care for people having dementia. Her activism includes visiting memory-care residences, some of which she says seem like dementia prisons. She calls for people living with dementia to audit care residences to determine whether staff members are enabling strengths, supporting individuality, and showing empathy.

Like Richard Taylor, Bryden is critical of how organizations raising money primarily for biomedical research do so by emphasizing the tragedy narrative to support their scare tactics. Reviewing a documentary film by the US Alzheimer's Association shown on public television in 2017, Dr. Bill Thomas quoted Bryden, who said:

> What causes the stigma and fear? It's the stereotype of dementia: someone who cannot understand, remembers nothing, and is unaware of what is happening around them. This stereotype tugs at the heartstrings and loosens the purse strings, so is used in seeking funds for research, support, and services. It's a catch 22, because Alzheimer's associations promote our image as non-persons, and make the stigma worse.[8]

In her book *What the Hell Happened to My Brain? Living Beyond Dementia*,[9] Kate Swaffer, also from Australia, recommends advocacy as an "intervention" for dementia. Other interventions she cites include blogging and volunteering. This is interesting, because most of the time people associate interventions for individuals living with dementia as pharmaceutical (such as the dangerous use of psychotropic drugs to deal with so-called "problem" behaviors[10]) or other types of therapies with scientifically sound evidence supporting their effectiveness. Often the person with dementia is a passive recipient of these interventions, with no choice in accepting them. For Swaffer, viewing advocacy as a kind of intervention attributes agency to the person with dementia.

Swaffer has little patience with organizations that claim to be promoting dementia-friendliness without consulting with people who actually have a type of dementia. She urges recognition of the fact that some with dementia do not want their condition advertised to the world. For example, she objects to installing "dementia lanes" in supermarkets, saying that stores would never have a "mental illness lane" or an "AIDS lane." Moreover, she thinks that people use the word "friend" in a facile way. She wants more meaningful engagement opportunities in dementia-enabling environments that support authentic relationships among friends, some of whom have a dementia. However, she does not want genuine human connection to be used merely as a marketing tool for organizations. In fact, she ends her book with this pithy observation: "There is, after all, big money in dementia."[11]

Taylor, Rohra, Bryden, and Swaffer may have stepped up to some of the earliest and most visible podiums for articulating their commitments to advocacy and activism, but many others are joining them in the effort to change dementia attitudes. Attitudes include beliefs, feelings, and actions, with actions often being a direct expression of what people believe about dementia and how they feel about the condition and the people living with its various symptoms. For better or for worse, these beliefs and feelings can shape the actions of family care-partners, friends, and professional caregivers.

Courageous people around the world are heeding Swaffer's call for advocacy and activism in the service of changing dementia attitudes. To support these efforts, Taylor had worked with Alzheimer's Disease International to develop a website to enable people to speak up and out. Called "I can! I will!" and designed as an idea library, the website contains advice on a variety of topics—including advocacy and activism—by people with dementia, care partners, medical professionals, professional carers, and Alzheimer's associations. Unfortunately, the website is no longer being updated, but the project's title and its archived material demonstrate the enthusiasm of people having dementia for telling their stories and encouraging others to take up the cause of changing dementia attitudes.[12]

Even though "I can! I will!" stopped accepting posts after Taylor's death, many other websites have arisen for people who wish to identify their priorities for governments, researchers, and for-profit and not-for-profit organizations. These online resources support the social citizenship of people living with dementia and serve as portals for them to spread their message about wanting to remain engaged with their communities and to battle the stereotypes attached to their condition. (Such stereotypes, it should be noted, often appear in messages from organizations focused on finding a dementia cure.) Writing about the online advocacy and activism of people living with dementia, historian Jesse Ballenger wrote this in a 2008 editorial in *Newsday*:

> Most of their effort supports the Alzheimer's movement's agenda of winning more public funding for research. But their activism also aims to battle stereotypical representations that Alzheimer's activists themselves have long used to make the case for funding—that people with dementia are no longer "really there," are no longer the person they once were, no longer even a person at all, having in effect already died, despite the troubling persistence of an animate body.[13]

Despite critiques by people having dementia like Christine Bryden, and of allies like Jesse Ballenger, many organizations around the world raise money for dementia research with the primary focus on cure and prevention. The promise of cure is both enticing and elusive, leaving some family members and friends in the uncomfortable position of supporting organizations primarily focused on cure while they struggle daily with lack of local support for coping with the challenges of living with dementia. Showing the fine line people like this walk, a friend who served on our regional Alzheimer's Association board and raised thousands of dollars for its coffers gave me permission to quote a statement he posted to his Facebook page:

> Wonderful advocacy work is being accomplished by the Alzheimer's Association in obtaining federal funding for research to hopefully find a cure for Alzheimer's. A worthy goal. However, what are we

learning from all the research? The number of people with dementia/ Alzheimer's continues to increase, and we have not yet found a way to slow or stop the progression. Hundreds of millions of dollars are spent on research, and yet the hundreds of millions of dollars in uncompensated care continue to rise. I would like to see an equal portion of funding go to both research and the cost of care. I facilitate three men's support groups, and many of us have been caring for our wives for years—in my case 10 years. We have raised money for the Alzheimer's Association, and we all agree that we would like to see the benefit of that fundraising support the cost of care in addition to research.

My friend and participants in his men's support groups organized a team for a fundraiser called Walking for Our Wives. They not only raise money but also advocate for greater awareness about the challenges men experience when caring for wives with some type of dementia. In addition, because of their experiences when their wives had to be hospitalized, they also advocate for the right to the compassionate medical care that many of them believe was denied their wives.

Human Rights and Dementia

Prompted in part by the activism and advocacy efforts of people having dementia, Scotland was the first country to develop a policy statement that reflects the United Nations Convention on the Rights of Persons with Disabilities. Scotland's "Charter of Rights for People with Dementia and their Carers" is meant for "people with dementia and their carers, at every stage of the illness and wherever they are."[14] Their policy statement is notable because it does not split those in the early phases of dementia from those whose dementia has progressed further. It also recognizes that people with dementia live in relationship with others. Scotland deliberately used an approach from the United Nations called PANEL, which affirms the rights of everyone living with dementia to the following:

- **Participation** in decisions that affect them, in access to community activities, in assessments about care needs, and in development of policies that affect them.

- Accountability by health and social-care professionals who have been trained in the human rights of persons living with dementia.

- Non-discrimination and equal treatment regardless of age, disability, gender, race, sexual orientation, religious beliefs, and social or other status.

- Empowerment to know their rights for full inclusion in decisions about their lives and to obtain the best possible physical and mental health care.

- Legality of all decisions and having these decisions grounded in respect for, and protection of, their human rights.[15]

The social model of dementia is gaining traction around the world as more people with the diagnosis and their care partners speak up for themselves. The social model considers the effects of the physical and the psychosocial environment on how persons living with dementia experience their worlds. It does not deny that identifiable changes occur in the brains of people with dementia symptoms. Activists such as those described in this chapter all acknowledge the difficulties they endure because of these brain changes. However, instead of focusing solely on the person whose brain is changing, the social model views persons having dementia within the context of their relationships with others and the places they live, love, work, and play. It affirms their dignity and the need to honor and protect their human rights. A newly published book on dementia and human rights states that achieving this requires that

- the voice of the person with dementia be heard

- service providers receive high-quality training

- public policy be reframed

- an intersectoral approach be adopted whereby change at an international level is driven by strong political leadership.[16]

No one should think that affirming human rights sugarcoats the experience of having dementia or caring for someone who has a dementia. Nor should anyone think that striving to create dementia-friendly communities is a simple matter of getting some interested people together to start a memory café. This work is hard. People who do not want to pay for needed programs and services will resist these efforts. Public-policy changes take time and often result in compromises disappointing to activists and advocates. Political leadership favoring dementia-friendly policies can be replaced with leadership having very different priorities. Nevertheless, despite challenges like these, people all over the world are working to promote quality of life, change the culture that excludes and stigmatizes people with dementia, and offer an array of options to support the social citizenship and human rights of people living with this progressive condition.

The Pluses and Minuses of Campaigning for Social Change

Being an agent of social change is not easy, but it can bring unexpected rewards. Ruth Bartlett, the researcher who coauthored the book *Broadening the Dementia Debate: Toward Social Citizenship*, learned this when she conducted a study of activism by people diagnosed with dementia. They described their activism in written diaries, photographs, and audio-diaries. Bartlett also interviewed them before and after they started keeping the diaries. Their activism took several forms, including speaking at conferences, lobbying politicians, and giving talks to students. According to Bartlett, they did this because they "wanted people with dementia to be treated fairly and as equal (rather than second-class) citizens."[17]

The participants in Bartlett's study knew that their cognitive abilities would decline, and this gave them a sense of urgency about their activism. Some of them felt that their work was a kind of health-promoting intervention, just as Kate Swaffer had asserted. The slogan "Use it or lose it" motivated many of them to work for change in policies and practices affecting people with dementia, and a few had doctors who supported the belief that their activities slowed the progression of their dementia symptoms. They also believed that their activism helped them retain a feeling of self-respect while also supporting their goal of encouraging respect for others with dementia. Another positive outcome was that they experienced a status boost from interacting with people in positions of power in the government or in dementia-advocacy organizations such as the Alzheimer's Society in the United Kingdom. Their activism resulted in making new friends, establishing social networks with other dementia activists, and expanding their vision of whom they might help. One man said, "I'm not gonna sit and let people walk over us. I'm going to stand up for people who won't talk or can't talk."[18]

One of the papers Bartlett wrote about this study documented some of what she called the "backstage" effects of being a dementia activist. For example, some of her participants described how they could give a rousing speech, but afterwards they would collapse with exhaustion. They also noted how tiring it was to write anything, including the diaries they were keeping for Bartlett. One man who submitted a photo-diary expressed his exhaustion by including a picture of himself sprawled on a sofa. They spoke not only of physical exhaustion but also of emotional exhaustion from putting themselves and their dementia symptoms on public display. A few expressed frustration with having their "illness credentials" questioned when people told them they looked and sounded so good. Occasionally, they felt exploited by powerful organizations. One woman said, "I feel, like others, that we are 'wheeled out' when needed."[19]

Everyone who participated in Bartlett's research knew they had limited time for speech-giving, letter-writing, and other dementia advocacy and activist work. So what happens when they can no longer speak for themselves? Although people living with advanced dementia in long-term-care settings can still be included in advocacy and activism, it is unlikely they will travel to conferences or write speeches. Who will SPEAK UP and OUT for them? Recall that Taylor borrowed that exhortation from observing how friends of people with AIDS had taken up the cause of urging more research and better care when the disease's progression and ultimate conclusion had rendered advocacy and activism impossible.

The next three chapters attempt to answer the question of who will speak for us when we can no longer speak for ourselves. Chapter 6 addresses the role of friendships in adding meaning and quality to the lives of people with dementia and their care partners. Like Taylor said, friends can also advocate for those no longer able to do it for themselves. Chapters 7 and 8 expand that discussion to communities committed to ensuring that the rights of persons with dementia are honored and that physical and psychosocial aspects of the community enable people to live as well as possible with this progressive condition. Those two chapters move the discussion from a focus on individual advocacy and activism to the work of organizations seeking changes in governmental policies and practices that support dementia-friendly community ideals.

Because this chapter began by describing Richard Taylor's advocacy and activism, I will give him the last word. This statement appeared in his very last newsletter. Though not denying that it would be wonderful to be able to halt dementia progression or even to eliminate its symptoms through biomedical research, Taylor asserted that much work could be done in communities that would more quickly yield beneficial results. He said:

> What we already have to work with are our communities. While readiness varies greatly between governmental entities, citizen-support services, and an aging and aged psycho-social infrastructure, these services can be, should be, our first respondents to this crisis. Our communities aren't just the best vehicles to work with, to strengthen, to fine tune, they are our only tools to realistically deal with the inevitability of this growing segment of everyone's population.

Dementia does not discriminate. In our increasingly polarized world, some people have become hesitant to state opinions about matters that could have political implications (for example, the need for more funding for respite care). However, dementia enters our lives without regard to political positions, and it ought to be one topic upon which people can find common ground. For example, I do not doubt that Republicans and Democrats in the United States love their parents, spouses, partners, and friends equally. When those loved ones begin the journey into dementia, together, with one voice, they should be able to SPEAK UP and OUT.

Endnotes

1 Taylor, R. (2007). *Alzheimer's from the inside out*. Baltimore, MD: Health Professions Press. (p. 244)

2 Taylor, p. 244.

3 Taylor, p. 244.

4 Unfortunately, I cannot give a citation for this quote from Richard Taylor's e-newsletter. Long before I had the idea of writing this book, I archived the emails containing the newsletter. Returning to them periodically reminds me of his tremendous courage and tenacity, as well as his sense of humor, as he tirelessly advocated for better lives for people having dementia.

5 Taylor, p. 68.

6 Rohra, H. (2016). *Dementia activist: Fighting for our rights*. London, UK: Jessica Kingsley Publishers.

7 Bryden, C. (2015). *Nothing about us without us: 20 years of dementia advocacy*. London, UK: Jessica Kingsley Publishers.

8 https://changingaging.org/dementia/every-person-counts

9 Swaffer, K. (2016). *What the hell happened to my brain? Living beyond dementia*. Philadelphia, PA: Jessica Kingsley Publishers.

10 Power, G. A. (2010). *Dementia beyond drugs: Changing the culture of care*. Baltimore, MD: Health Professions Press.

11 Swaffer, p. 341.

12 https://icaniwill.alz.co.uk/icaniwill.html

13 Ballenger's editorial was published online on July 20, 2008. Unfortunately, it no longer appears to be available.
    Ballenger, J. (2008, July 20). Alzheimer's patients need to be engaged citizens [Editorial]. *Newsday*.

14 Alzheimer Scotland. (2009). *Charter of rights for people with dementia and their carers in Scotland*. Edinburgh, UK: Alzheimer Scotland, p. 5. Accessed on 7/22/19 at www.alzscot.org/assets/0000/2678/Charter_of_Rights.pdf

15 Alzheimer Scotland, p. 4.

16 Cahill, S. (2018). *Dementia and human rights*. Chicago, IL: Policy Press. (p. 9)

17 Bartlett, R. (2014). The emergent modes of dementia activism. *Aging & Society, 34*, 623–644. (p. 632)

18 Bartlett, p. 637.

19 Bartlett, R. (2014). Citizenship in action: The lived experiences of citizens with dementia who campaign for social change. *Disability & Society, 29*, 1291–1304. (p. 1300)

Part 3

FRIENDSHIP AND COMMUNITY INCLUSION

Chapter 6

Accompanying Friends Through the Journey of Dementia

Suzy and Grace have been friends since junior high. Now they are in their mid-50s and have come to their first memory café. As they enter a room full of people sitting around tables in a library meeting room, they laughingly describe how their friendship goes back to the time of young-teen hijinks.

Suzy is learning to live with younger-onset Alzheimer's disease, and Grace has promised to accompany her through the "strange land" of dementia.[1] They do not know what to expect at a memory café but have heard that it is a time set aside for enjoying camaraderie, coffee, sweet treats, and some kind of engaging program without the stigma usually attached to a dementia diagnosis. (Chapter 8 includes information about starting and operating memory cafés.)

As I greet them and write out their nametags, I think about how unusual it is for friends to enjoy memory cafés together. Most of the time, memory café participants attend with their spouses, partners, adult children, or siblings. It is rare for friends to come to memory cafés. However, memory cafés provide a marvelous opportunity for friends to share an enjoyable experience while giving family care-partners respite for a couple of hours.

The memory café regulars greet Suzy and Grace warmly, and a few minutes after everyone gathers, we sing our welcoming song, naming each person in the room. Everyone smiles and waves to the group as their names are sung, and I can see that Suzy and Grace appear to be comfortably settled into this new experience.[2]

Although Suzy and Grace have known each other for decades, a number of other friendships in the room are relatively new, formed among people who regularly attend memory cafés. Some also participate in day-long bus trips that include lunch and visits to local attractions, gather at monthly informal "meet-ups" at a family restaurant, and sing together in a chorus that performs at local venues.[3] None of these activities are unusual for friends to enjoy together, but these are people living with a condition often associated with social isolation and loneliness, both for the diagnosed person and the care partner.

How do I know about these new friendships? Memory-café participants tell me that they have exchanged phone numbers and email addresses. They describe how couples invite other couples to their homes for supper. Several widows continue to attend memory cafés, participate in outings, sing in the chorus, and meet for weekly card games. They forged important relationships while caring for their husbands who had dementia. In other words, we can think of memory cafés as friendship incubators.

The friendship of Suzy and Grace was incubated in the hallways and after-school activities of junior high. Now they are experiencing the resilience of that relationship as it is tested by Suzy's dementia. For now, it appears that Grace is committed to learning her way into this new form of friendship that involves coming to a library on a Monday afternoon to gather with people living with dementia as diagnosed persons and care partners. What will happen to their friendship when Suzy can no longer remember the stories of their younger selves? How does Grace feel about the way dementia is shifting the contours of their friendship? Will Grace visit Suzy if Suzy's husband can no longer care for her in their home and she needs to relocate to a memory-care community? I have no definite answers to these questions, but I am hopeful that community programs like memory cafés can support friendships like theirs.

This chapter asserts that much can be learned about friendship from Suzy and Grace, from the memory-café participants forming new relationships, and from people having dementia who live in some type of long-term-care community. There is a lot of talk these days about dementia-friendly communities, but what does the "friend" part of that label really mean?

What Is a Friend?

A few years ago, my husband and I wrote a book about friendship, dementia, and flourishing communities.[4] We noted that gerontologists who studied aging had not spent much time looking into friendships; their attention to social interactions centered on families. When studying people living with dementia, researchers' field of view became even narrower as they focused on individuals and their brains.

In our attempt to grasp the meaning of friendship, we found it helpful to review what Aristotle had to say over two thousand years ago. He noted that some friendships are based on what people can do for one another (friendships based on utility) and some derive from the enjoyment people share (friendships based on pleasure). Aristotle described these two types of friendship as incomplete because friendships can end when people feel they no longer benefit their friends or give them pleasure.[5] A third type of friendship, Aristotle argued, is based on virtue: friends share joys and sorrows while trying to help one another lead good and virtuous lives. He called these friendships complete and said that people experiencing virtuous friendships commit to spending time with one another.

Interestingly, soon after we wrote our book and noted how little attention had been paid to friendship and dementia, an entire issue of the journal *Dementia: The International Journal of Social Research and Practice* was given over to nine articles about friendship. In one paper, Phyllis Braudy Harris reported on interviews she conducted with people in the early stages of dementia. The descriptions and definitions of friendships she heard in these interviews resemble those offered by Aristotle.

Harris's research participants told her that friendships were important to them because they felt comfortable with their friends and trusted them. They could be honest with friends because they felt understood and accepted. One woman described the way in which she continues to maintain utility in a friendship:

When I go out to lunch or for coffee with my friend, it is important to me that I pay my share; we take turns paying. Now, I don't remember, but I know I can trust my friend to tell me when it is my turn. I know she wants to pick up the tab, but she knows how important it is to me.[6]

Harris also heard many stories about friendships based on pleasure. Importantly, the research participants said that their friends could look beyond their cognitive disability. For example, another woman told Harris:

I'm still active, and I'm in a golf league, and I get worse and worse every year, and the girls in the league won't let me quit. They say I am a role model.[7]

One theme Harris extracted from the interviews aligns with Aristotle's reflections on complete, virtuous friendship: friends share core values and help people living with dementia to maintain their values. One person talked about how much she values her independence even if tasks take her longer to accomplish and are harder for her than for most people. She said that her friend understands and respects this desire. Another woman described how she has always been someone who wants to take care of others. Now she has a friend with whom she delivers Meals on Wheels, and together they enjoy a shared, valued activity.

Why Friends Matter

In 2018, the insurance company Cigna released a report on loneliness in the United States based on a survey of twenty thousand Americans. The data showed that loneliness presents a greater risk to health than obesity or smoking. Using a comparison that quickly gained traction in news reports and on social media, the company's chief medical officer asserted that loneliness has the same effect on mortality as smoking 15 cigarettes a day.[8] Although I do not know of any scientific studies that actually tested this claim, even the US Health Resources and Services Administration reiterated it.[9] The same year the Cigna study came out, the United Kingdom appointed a Minister for Loneliness, recognizing that this is a problem not only for persons with dementia and their care partners, and not only for elders living alone, but also for young people, people with disabilities, refugees, and others who feel isolated even when in physical contact with people.

Artists, writers, and musicians have often depicted the human need for companionship and the effects on the human mind, body, and spirit when it is absent. As the last century drew to a close, scientists began examining the effects of social relationships on a long list of health outcomes. In 1988, one of the world's premier science journals published an article summarizing the literature on a *causal* relationship between the quality and quantity of social relationships and various health measures. At the end of their article, the authors looked ahead to the twenty-first century, noting that in the 1970s, American adults "were less likely to be married, more likely to be living alone, less likely to belong to voluntary organizations, and less likely to visit informally with others."[10] They worried that the mounting evidence about the impact of social relationships on health coincided with the demographics of aging, and they predicted that many older persons would lack the support from family members and friends offered to previous generations of older people.

One health outcome not mentioned in the 1988 paper on social relationships and health was dementia. This connection was addressed in the first decade of this century when three widely cited longitudinal studies concluded that having a higher level of social integration may have a protective effect against dementia.[11] A number of possible reasons for this have been suggested. For example, perhaps having contact with more people motivates individuals to take better care of themselves in terms of diet and exercise. Social interactions may offer cognitive stimulation that could build cognitive reserve. More social connections could even give people a greater sense of purpose in life. None of these factors function like a vaccine against types of dementia, but by reducing stress and supporting cardiovascular health, they could have a positive effect on brain health.

Around the same time these papers on social relationships and dementia appeared, researchers and policy makers in many countries began to pay more attention to the number of older people living alone with shrinking social networks. Of course, living alone does not necessarily predict the emotional response of loneliness. For example, one large study in the Netherlands followed socially isolated older people for three years. They lived alone, were unmarried, and had no social support. These factors by themselves did not predict a higher dementia risk. The authors stated that it was "not the objective situation [of living alone] but rather the perceived absence of social attachments that increases the risk of cognitive decline."[12] In other words, it was the loneliness that raised the dementia risk.

Loneliness is stressful. A large Australian study of people with dementia and family care-partners suggested that

> loneliness might compromise neural systems underlying cognition and memory, which in turn might make lonely individuals more vulnerable to deleterious effects of age-related neuropathology by decreasing neural reserve.[13]

In this study, the care partners felt lonely, too. Some of them talked about the social stigma attached not only to dementia but also to loneliness. In addition, both care partners and their loved ones with dementia often had other chronic health issues that limited their ability to stay connected to other people. Mobility challenges limited their social contacts, and hearing loss affected their social engagement. One man said that he had stopped going to a local recreation hall "because now that my hearing is gone, that has restricted an awful lot of social life that I used to have."[14]

Friends matter. What human beings have always intuited about their need for social relationships now has plenty of supportive scientific evidence. People living with a dementia—as diagnosed persons and care partners—know that friends matter. When they are asked about the key components of living well with dementia, relationships rise to the top of their lists.[15] However, they also describe how their old friends drift away and how hard it is to make new friends. That is the often-told story about friendship and dementia. But that is also the story that Suzy and Grace are challenging.

Accompaniment

Grace's accompaniment of Suzy takes two forms. In the usual way we think of accompaniment, Grace brings Suzy to memory cafés. They literally walk side by side as they come into the public library. However, there is another form of accompaniment that is less obvious but just as important: psychosocial accompaniment. Grace's commitment to bringing Suzy to memory cafés can be interpreted as openness to accompanying Suzy on her journey "through change, loss, frailty, and limits."[16] Some people understand this accompaniment as spiritual as well as psychosocial.

That quote about accompaniment comes from my longtime friend, Rabbi Dayle Friedman, author of many books and papers about being present to elders, especially frail elders with some type of dementia. Writing about Jewish pastoral care, Rabbi Friedman says that rabbinic accompaniment, or *livui ruchani* in Hebrew, means walking "along with people through the sorrows, joys, and everyday moments of their lives."[17]

Of course, we do not need to be rabbis to do this for our friends, nor do we have to see these acts as spiritual. However, as Rabbi Friedman writes, we do need humility and respect. We need humility to acknowledge that we could be the ones having a dementia who need our friends to remain fully present to us. Humility comes from acknowledging our own vulnerability and our own fears of aging and dementia. Respect for our friends is essential in this journey of accompaniment, for we must always treat them as the adults they are and adapt our interactions with them to accommodate their needs (for example, by slowing down).

Old Friends

I recently chatted with an older woman at a community fundraising event. When I told her about writing this book, she got a pained expression on her face and described a longtime friend who may have some type of dementia. This woman said that her friend asks her a question and then repeats the question 10 minutes later. I sympathized with her distress over the change in her friend and suggested that she might gently suggest that her friend talk with her doctor about memory concerns. I also said that if the friend eventually does receive a dementia diagnosis, then it will be critically important for her to promise to accompany her friend regardless of where the dementia journey takes her. The woman looked troubled by what I said, so I did not press her to say more. Given the social setting where this conversation took place, I did not have an opportunity to pursue the conversation. If I had, I would have talked about how people can learn new and meaningful ways to remain close to their friends living with dementia.

It is hard for friends to engage in difficult conversations such as suggesting the possibility of an assessment when a friend shows worrisome signs of forgetfulness. Friendships grounded solely in utility or pleasure may not be able to accommodate such conversations. However, a virtuous friendship, which means we want what is good for our friend, might require that we take the risk of talking about our concerns about our friend's memory lapses and confusion.

Similarly, Janelle Taylor, an anthropologist at the University of Toronto, talks about people who find ways to remain in friendship with a person having dementia, no matter how difficult it may be. She calls such people "exemplary friends." In her research, she has begun to interview friends like this in order to learn what motivates them, frustrates them, and gratifies them. She has discovered that some people are able to rise to the moral challenge of not turning away from someone who has developed dementia symptoms and to accept the new story that has been inserted into the longtime friendship. Grace's accompaniment of Suzy puts her in this category.

The exemplary friends who have talked with Taylor know that they are doing something unusual, because they see others who have ended relationships with their friends with dementia. Some of these exemplary friends collaborate with mutual friends so that together they can establish a course of action to assist the family care-partner (if there is one) and to continue the relationship with the person having dementia.

Such collaboration usually requires talking with one another about the person with dementia—sharing notes about how the visits have been going and what the person with dementia seems to need and enjoy. This may bring up the question, Does such note-sharing count as gossip? We usually think of gossip as mean-spirited, but Taylor has a different way of looking at this kind of talking and sharing. She prefers to consider "the possibility that dementia might be met collectively and with love and joy."[18] When conversations take the form of "How can we help our friend and her care partner?" they cannot be called gossip. They are motivated by love and rewarded with joy.

Taylor offers a beautiful metaphor inspired by the book and film *Still Alice*. Those who have read the book may recall that an image of a butterfly appears on its cover and that butterflies flutter through several pages in the book. Taylor says that friends who come together to accompany someone with dementia create a cocoon for the friend:

> Through rising to meet the challenges presented by dementia, a group can make or remake itself as a moral community and offer itself to vulnerable members as a "cocoon"—in other words, a safe place within which to undergo a transformation.[19]

The transformation in a longtime friendship will not always be smooth, and it will certainly include sadness and loss. However, accompanying a friend through the changes can also offer opportunities for growth and unexpected joy.

Becoming an Exemplary Friend

As a person negotiates a changing relationship with a friend with dementia, some practical tips can be helpful. Dementia advocacy organizations in Australia[20] and Scotland[21] offer a number of suggestions, which I have summarized here:

- Friends need to educate themselves about dementia and avoid touting "snake oil remedies" with no proven efficacy.

- Friends should learn to not take things personally. Sometimes the person with dementia is having a bad day and may not want to visit. Being aware of triggers for mood swings becomes important in some relationships.

- As the friend's dementia progresses, it's helpful to practice "redirecting" the friend's attention if they become anxiously focused on one concern. For example, a person might repeatedly ask if it is time to go for a doctor's appointment that has already happened or will happen in the future. A friend might reply, "I know you're eager to see your doctor, but let's take a few minutes to go look at the flowers in that garden."

- It is important to slow down in speaking and physical movements, because it may take the person longer to process verbal information, and because the individual's balance and mobility may be affected by the dementia.

- Friends should not offer too many choices, because that can be overwhelming. If the person with dementia is scanning a restaurant menu, for example, instead of saying "What looks good to you?" think of what types of food they normally enjoy and then say, "Would you like the cheeseburger or the chicken salad?"

- Persons living with dementia can feel shame or distress when others try to correct their perceptions or memory lapses. Friends need to learn to "go with the flow" of conversations. And while people disagree about the morality of white lies, many dementia care-partners find such an approach more compassionate than repeatedly reminding a person of a fact that will upset them. For example, if a man living with the middle or late stage of dementia says "Where is my wife?" his friend can reply that she will be coming home from work in a few hours, not that she died.

- Friends should be sensitive about avoiding environments that may be too stimulating for someone having dementia.

- Friends need to be patient. Joy Watson, a woman who has lived with Alzheimer's dementia for two years, wrote in an editorial in the journal *Dementia*: "People haven't always got the patience to listen while it takes you ages to complete a sentence. I've learned to read people's body language, so usually I know when they are eager to get away."[22]

Watson's point about body language is worth noting. People with dementia often appear to have a sixth sense for nonverbal emotion cues. Greeting a person with a fake smile and a too-cheery demeanor can quickly derail a visit. It's helpful to relax and to slow down.

Friends of people having dementia sometimes rationalize their decision not to engage in the tasks of accompaniment by saying that their friend cannot remember their interactions so it is pointless to make the effort. This is wrong, and scientists who study emotion agree. The positive feelings engendered by a pleasant interaction with a friend can last long after the visit ends. Think about it! When we feel happy, all kinds of good neurological responses are coursing through our brains. In a book about the physiology of love, the three authors (all physicians) offer one of my favorite pithy statements reflecting this research: "A relationship *is* a physiologic process, as real and as potent as any pill or surgical procedure."[23]

A similar statement was offered by Danny George, a medical anthropologist, and Peter Whitehouse, a neurologist, who spent many years working on some of the early Alzheimer's dementia drugs. They wrote:

> We believe that every psychosocial intervention is also de facto a biological intervention. Telling a story, reading a book, or participating in talk therapy engenders complex but undoubtedly real changes in the brain. In fact, it is not a stretch to refer to reading a book as a multineurotransmitter, neuroprotective, lexical access enhancement device, especially when pills tend to act on only one or just a few primary neurotransmitter systems![24]

If a person with dementia can feel the love expressed when interacting with a friend, and those good feelings last for a while after the visit ends, then does it really matter if the person cannot remember the friend's name, what they did together, or the story of their friendship?

Janelle Taylor, who researched and wrote about exemplary friends, also wrote about her mother's advanced dementia. She observed that people repeatedly posed this question: "Does she recognize you?" We have all heard stories about people having dementia not recognizing their family members. Taylor said that her mother was always happy to see her but that it had been years since her mom spoke her name. Sometimes her mother called her "Stranger," but she did so in an affectionate way.

Apparently, most of Taylor's mother's friends could not cope with the changes brought by her dementia. Taylor wrote to these friends when her mom relocated to a dementia-care community and suggested how much she would enjoy hearing from them. No one responded! Taylor concluded that many of these friendships had been based on pleasure and could not "bear the weight of deep and diffuse obligations to care… Dementia seems to act as a very powerful solvent on many kinds of social ties."[25]

Taylor discovered what many exemplary friends know: even if a friend no longer remembers you or your friendship, a visit can be pleasant with lasting good feelings for both the person with dementia and the friend. She described the deep and satisfying sense of being "in the moment" while interacting with her mother. Together they sat and enjoyed watching puffy white clouds on a summer day; they walked hand in hand around the memory-care community and noticed small, delightful details like someone's blue sweater or a child's laugh. In this ordinary interaction, they shared wonder and joy, which then became a satisfying, meaningful way of communicating. Taylor's mother may not have recognized her in our usual way of thinking about recognition, but at a deeper level, Taylor knew that her mother cared about her. For her mother, caring was a deeply ingrained habit that she drew upon repeatedly when interacting with people whose names she no longer recalled.

New Friends

Sometimes people with dementia and care partners make new friends after the diagnosis. As I mentioned earlier, I see this happen all the time at memory cafés, on bus trips, at informal meet-ups for supper at local restaurants, and in the relationships formed among members of the chorus I coordinate.[26] These friendships develop as people share enjoyable interactions in spaces where no one needs to apologize for forgetfulness, confusion, loss of language, or the other behavioral expressions so common to dementia.

Once, on a daylong bus trip that included lunch in a restaurant's private dining room, I sat next to a man who quickly ate the piece of cake included with his place setting. On any other dining occasion, his wife might have admonished him for eating dessert first. On that day, she knew she did not have to be embarrassed, because they were with a group that understood the impulses—and love of sweets—

of many people living with dementia. Important and lasting bonds form as a result of this openness and acceptance.

New friendships can emerge informally from shared activities such as memory cafés. They can also happen as a result of frequent interactions with strangers who become friends in a variety of settings. For example, my husband has a longtime friend who now lives with Parkinson's disease and vascular dementia. His friend can no longer drive, so about every three weeks, my husband takes his friend for lunch at a restaurant called Draft Gastropub. It is a very busy place where a lot of business people dash in for quick lunches. The manager of the restaurant and several of the wait staff now recognize them, lead them to a quiet table, and happily serve the friend lobster bisque and lobster pie, the meal he orders every time. No one says it is odd for one person to have so much lobster while the other person has a simple salad or sandwich. They are encouraged to stay as long as they want. They take turns paying the bill with their credit cards, but no one comments on how my husband has to calculate the tip.

Both my husband and his friend feel comfortable and welcome there, especially because the manager and servers have learned their names. In other words, the restaurant employees see my husband's friend as a person, not as someone whose gait is unusual and who appears unable to read a menu or figure out a tip.

The people working at Draft Gastropub are behaving like dementia friends. I use the phrase "dementia friends" deliberately, because that is the name of an international movement to train people to be new friends of people having dementia. In 2013, the Alzheimer's Society in the UK began the Dementia Friends program as a way of teaching people about dementia, reducing stigma, and encouraging the development of dementia-friendly communities.[27] Becoming a Dementia Friend requires just a few hours of time for an in-person training or watching a video, along with a pledge to do better at reaching out to connect helpfully with people having dementia. This could be a neighbor or a person working in a drugstore, bank, post office, or a place like the restaurant where my husband and his friend go. The basic idea is to lay the groundwork for dementia-friendly communities by establishing social relationships. The program has spread quickly and is now promoted in the US by the nonprofit organization Dementia Friendly America (DFA), which offers online videos to train Dementia Friends and also licenses statewide organizations to provide classroom Dementia Friends training.[28]

The new friendships I have observed at memory cafés and other programs in my community, as well as the comfortable and welcoming interactions enjoyed by my husband and his friend, were formed informally. No one instructed these people in dementia friendliness. But formal training in dementia friendliness such as that offered by DFA has begun to happen in places like high schools and colleges with service-learning requirements. In Wisconsin, the Department of Health Services developed a curriculum on dementia for high-school students that can be incorporated into required health classes. Students have the option of taking the Dementia Friends training and volunteering for regular visits in a local long-term-care community.

Some undergraduate and graduate programs in the health professions assign students to meet regularly with a person with dementia. For example, at the Mailman School of Public Health at Columbia University, a program called "A Friend for Rachel" has been offered for seven years. Students studying for various health professions commit to seeing someone with mild to moderate dementia once a week for a year. They also participate in eight trainings through the year and write weekly reflections about their visits. In one story told by Dr. Jill Goldman,[29] director of the program, a very shy pre-med student was matched with a woman in her early 50s with primary progressive aphasia who could no longer speak. It turned out that the student was also a dancer. She learned to communicate with her new friend through gestures and movements. Dr. Goldman reports that about 35 percent of the students remain in relationship with their friends for two to three years.[30]

Of course, students graduate and move on in their lives, so these new friendships may not endure. Other formal programs have more success in nurturing friendships that last longer. The best examples may come from faith communities (described in Chapter 10) that offer training about dementia and connections to people living with it. Usually they have periodic meetings for the new friends to receive additional training and share insights about being a friend with people having dementia and their care partners. Sometimes these friendship-training programs are described as a formal way of promoting "facilitated friendship."

Facilitating Friendships

Although friendships can be facilitated—that is, encouraged and strengthened—by such programs hosted by high schools, colleges and universities, and faith communities, friendship is more often facilitated in an informal manner. A person with dementia can feel more comfortable and social in some physical spaces and in some groups than in others. Take the Draft Gastropub mentioned above, a busy restaurant catering mostly to people on their lunch breaks. One might not initially think of it as a place where a person with a type of dementia would feel comfortable. However, my husband and his friend interact easily with others and there is a quieter corner of the restaurant where they can settle in every time they go there. In other words, friendships are facilitated by a combination of the physical environment and the psychosocial characteristics of the people in that environment.

Another example comes from my friend Lucille. She needed to move her husband to our county skilled-nursing center when his dementia became too challenging for her to handle at home. Formerly the county asylum, it was rebuilt from the ground up about 20 years ago with what at that time was a radical new design for long-term care: a large building made up of small households organized into neighborhoods. About once a month, Lucille invited several friends to share a dinner with her and her husband in his new home. She brought tablecloths, electric candles, and delicious food, setting it all out in a small family room furnished with attractive tables and chairs and art on the walls. Together the friends enjoyed an evening of fellowship. Lucille facilitated the continuation of friendship by her meal planning and preparation, as well as her devotion to keeping her husband included in their longtime group of friends. The long-term-care community also had a role in that facilitation because it provided an attractive gathering place for friends.

Similar stories can be found in the admittedly sparse literature on friendships among persons living in long-term-care communities or participating in adult day services. One Australian study conducted in the secure memory-care unit of a nursing home noted that most of the events provided for the residents needing memory care involved passive entertainment for the whole group and offered little opportunity for interpersonal interaction.[31] Perhaps if the staff had received more training, and thus been more attuned to the importance of interpersonal relationships and ways to facilitate them, they might have taken a different approach to planning activities.

A different study done in Australia found that loneliness was not magically ameliorated just because people were seated at dining-room tables near one another.[32] The physical environment alone was not enough to facilitate socializing if staff did not create an atmosphere that invited pleasant interactions and the possibility for friendships to develop. For example, taking a few minutes for a creative-engagement activity before serving a meal could encourage residents to connect with one another in a meaningful, enjoyable way. Another study that specifically addressed the role of both the physical and the psychosocial environment in promoting social interaction among residents of a dementia-care community concluded that organizations with a less rigid hierarchy of staff roles seemed better able to support staff in encouraging informal social interaction. That research also examined social-interaction differences that arose based on the location of the nursing station. The researchers found that making the nursing station blend in with primary activity space encouraged staff–resident interactions as well as interactions among residents. In other words, residents' relational needs were best met when the physical environment was designed to meet these needs and when staff intentionally promoted relationality.[33]

Interviews and observations of people in dementia-care settings have resulted in many examples of residents helping one another. In one study, the researchers stated that it would be beneficial if staff noticed, reinforced, and promoted these expressions of "feelings of concern, love, nurturance, and support" shown by residents toward one another.[34] In my experience, most of the people who work in these kinds of care communities want their residents to have the best lives possible, including having meaningful relationships with other residents and staff. Unfortunately, too many of these employees are overworked, underpaid, and not respected for their knowledge about residents' strengths and needs. Their efforts to encourage friendships among residents may go unnoted and unrewarded.

Friendship and Community

Exemplary friends such as Grace reject the old story about how friends cut friendship ties once dementia symptoms emerge. It is not hard to see how that can happen if the friendship is grounded solely in utility or in pleasure. Grace's friendship with Suzy illustrates a virtuous, and an exemplary, friendship. However, we cannot ignore elements of utility and pleasure in their relationship. Yes, Grace brings Suzy to the memory café, but the pleasure they share is a gift returned to Grace. Suzy may no longer be able to help Grace in her garden or drive Grace's children to school, but I think that Grace would say that her effort to bring Suzy to the library is rewarded by Suzy's delight in the singing and socializing at the café. We should never forget the importance of shared fun in adult friendships, even when dementia enters the picture.

Dementia gets us down to basics. Accompanying our friends through dementia and discovering meaningful ways of remaining in relationship requires that we abandon the common bleak narratives about their condition as well as the defensive denial of the losses dementia brings to our lives. It is hard, but important, to learn to live with our sadness about the changes wrought by dementia while also remaining open to possibilities for love and joy in moments of connection with our friends.

Whether old or new, friendships do not exist in a vacuum. This obvious statement directs our attention to the importance of communities that support and sustain opportunities for friendship. If the community where Grace and Suzy live had no memory cafés, I do not know what their options might be for enjoying a pleasant afternoon together. Perhaps Grace might hear about memory cafés or similar programs and, thinking about Suzy, she might advocate for dementia-friendly efforts. Friends visiting a memory-care community and observing bored, lonely, and helpless people with dementia might advocate for better staff training and support for activities that encourage social ties through creative engagement.

Friends who take someone to a restaurant where servers ignore the person having dementia, speak too quickly, and offer too many options might advocate for dementia-friendly training in that business. Friends concerned about the lack of education about dementia in their communities might advocate in their state legislatures for programs to inform citizens about dementia.

When confronted by the current and predicted demographics of aging and dementia, some people want to hide their heads in the sand. These same people may find it impossible to sustain relationships when their friends develop dementia. Thankfully, there are others like Grace who courageously remain open to possibilities for continuing their friendship while grieving the changes their friends are experiencing. It is much easier to do this when a community honors the strengths and assets of people with dementia and their care partners. Together, people can encourage their communities to undertake the challenge of becoming dementia aware, capable, enabling, friendly, inclusive, positive, and supportive. Part of this effort should involve encouraging people to accompany their friends into the strange land of dementia and to discover the rewards of doing so. The next two chapters offer specific ideas about how communities might do this.

Endnotes

1   Malcolm Goldsmith was a beloved Anglican priest in Scotland. He served several parishes, worked as a hospice chaplain, and was a Research Fellow at the Dementia Services Development Centre at the University of Stirling. He wrote several books about serving people with dementia, including one that specifically focused on ministry. He called the book *In a Strange Land*: Goldsmith, M. (2004). *In a strange land: People with dementia and the local church*. Edinburgh, UK: MD Print & Design.

2   Memory cafés are programs, not places, although some memory café programs meet in actual cafés. Many libraries have launched memory café programs, and memory cafés can also be found in nature centers, museums, and other public spaces. Much information about starting and sustaining memory cafés can be found via internet searches. For example, here is a memory café toolkit from Wisconsin: McFadden, S. (2017). *Wisconsin memory café programs: A best practice guide*. Madison, WI: Wisconsin Alzheimer's Institute, University of Wisconsin School of Medicine and Public Health. Accessed on 7/2/20 at https://wai.wisc.edu/best-practice-guides

3   These and other similar social activities are programs of Fox Valley Memory Project, a nonprofit located in northeast Wisconsin: www.foxvalleymemoryproject. org/get-social

4   McFadden, S. H., & McFadden, J. T. (2011). *Aging together: Dementia, friendship, and flourishing communities*. Baltimore, MD: Johns Hopkins University Press.

5   This may be why so many people with dementia, along with their care partners, say their friends abandon them. Because care partners and diagnosed persons can become so consumed with the challenges of daily life, they or their friends may conclude that reciprocity in friendship is no longer possible. In addition, because of those challenges, people living with dementia may have to stop participating in the pleasurable activities they once enjoyed with their friends.

6   Harris, P. B. (2011). Maintaining friendships in early-stage dementia: Factors to consider. *Dementia, 11*, 305–314. (p. 309)

7   Harris, p. 311.

8   Nemecek, D. (2018). *Cigna U.S. loneliness index*. Bloomfield, CT: Cigna. Accessed on 7/29/18 at www.multivu.com/players/English/8294451-cigna-us-loneliness-survey/docs/IndexReport_1524069371598-173525450.pdf

9   An internet search for "loneliness and health" yields many scientific papers and media articles. The HRSA statement about 15 cigarettes a day appears at www.hrsa. gov/enews/past-issues/2019/january-17/loneliness-epidemic

10 House, J. S., Landis, K. R., & Umberson, D. (1988). Social relationships and health. *Science, 241*, 540–545. (p. 544)

11 Bennett, D. A., Schneider, J. A., Tang, Y., Arnold, S. E., & Wilson, R. S. (2006). The effect of social networks on the relation between Alzheimer's disease pathology and level of cognitive function in old people: A longitudinal cohort study. *The Lancet Neurology, 5*, 406–412.

Ertel, K. A., Glymour, M., & Berkman, L. F. (2008). Effects of social integration on preserving memory function in a nationally representative US elderly population. *American Journal of Public Health, 98*, 1215–1220.

Fratiglioni, L., Paillard-Borg, S., & Winblad, B. (2004). An active and socially integrated lifestyle in late life might protect against dementia. *The Lancet Neurology, 3*, 343–353.

12 Holwerda, T. J., Deeg, D. J. H., Beekman, A. T. F., van Tilburg, T. G., Stek, M. L., Jonker, C., et al. (2014). Feelings of loneliness, but not social isolation, predict dementia onset: Results from the Amsterdam Study of the Elderly (AMSTEL). *Journal of Neurology, Neurosurgery, and Psychiatry, 5*, 135–142. (p. 137)

13 Moyle, W., Kellett, U., Ballantyne, A., & Gracia, N. (2011). Dementia and loneliness: An Australian perspective. *Journal of Clinical Nursing, 20*, 1445–1453. (p. 1446)

14 Moyle et al., p. 1449. This plaintive comment highlights the need to address the relationship between hearing loss and dementia symptoms, not only because addressing hearing loss could delay or prevent dementia symptoms but also so that people already living with dementia do not experience excess disability due to their inability to hear and participate in social interaction.

15 Linda Clare, a British neuropsychologist mentioned in Chapter 2, is leading a major longitudinal research program in England to learn the factors related to living well with dementia. At the 2018 meeting of Alzheimer's Disease International, Dr. Clare stated that low levels of depression and loneliness were the strongest predictors. For more information about this study, see: www.idealproject.org.uk/people

16 Friedman, D. A. (2005). Letting their faces shine: Accompanying aging people and their families. In D. A. Friedman (Ed.), *Jewish pastoral care: A practical handbook*

from traditional and contemporary sources (2nd ed., pp. 344–373). Woodstock, VT: Jewish Lights Publishing. (p. 359)

17 Friedman, p. 359.

18 Taylor, J. S. (2017). Engaging with dementia: Moral experiments in art and friendship. *Culture, Medicine, and Psychiatry, 41,* 282–303. (p. 299)

19 Taylor, p. 300.

20 Alzheimer's Australia. (2012). *Friends matter: How to stay connected to a friend living with dementia.* Melbourne, Australia: Alzheimer's Australia. Accessed on 7/18/19 at www.dementia.org.au/sites/default/files/Friends_Matter_24pp_booklet_ with_checklist.pdf

21 Alzheimer Scotland. (2015). *"I'll get by with a little help from my friends": Information for friends of people with dementia.* Edinburgh, UK: Alzheimer Scotland. Accessed on 7/18/19 at www.alzscot.org/assets/0001/7435/Friends_Booklet_lo-res.pdf

22 Watson, J. (2016). Is it possible to live well with dementia? *Dementia, 15,* 4–5. (p. 5)

23 Lewis, T., Amini, F., & Lannon, R. (2000). *A general theory of love.* New York, NY: Vintage Books. (p. 81)

24 George, D., & Whitehouse, P. J. (2009). The classification of Alzheimer's disease and mild cognitive impairment: Enriching therapeutic models through moral imagination. In J. G. Ballenger, P. J. Whitehouse, C. G. Lyketsos, P. V. Rabins, & J. H. T. Karlawish (Eds.), *Treating dementia: Do we have a pill for it?* (pp. 5–24). Baltimore, MD: Johns Hopkins University Press. (p. 20)

25 This powerful reflection on recognition, written from the heart of a daughter accompanying her mother through advanced dementia, is worth the effort of asking a librarian for help in accessing it: Taylor, J. S. (2008). On recognition, caring, and dementia. *Medical Anthropology Quarterly, 22,* 313–335. (p. 319)

26 These are examples of programs offered by Fox Valley Memory Project: www. foxvalleymemoryproject.org

27 www.dementiafriends.org.uk

28 Dementia Friendly America (DFA) is licensed by the international Dementia Friends program developed by the Alzheimer's Society in the UK. Through its website, it offers online video training for Dementia Friends. States licensed by DFA can offer classroom training by Dementia Champions who have taken additional classes in order to become trainers: www.dfamerica.org

29 Personal communication, April 15, 2019. See also the Student Artists in Residence program at the University of Wisconsin–Milwaukee begun by Anne Basting, founder of TimeSlips (https://uwm.edu/community/students/student-artist-in-residence). TimeSlips offers training for high-school and college students and teachers in its evidence-based creative storytelling method and encourages students to commit to doing this in long-term-care settings for 8–10 weeks: www.timeslips. org

30 Goldman, J. S., & Trommer, A. E. (2019). A qualitative study of the impact of a dementia experiential learning project on pre-medical students: A friend for Rachel. *BMC Medical Education, 19*(127). Accessed on 4/14/20 at https:// bmcmededuc.biomedcentral.com/track/pdf/10.1186/s12909-019-1565-3

31 Casey, A-N. S., Low, L-F., Jeon, Y-H., & Brodaty, H. (2016). Residents' perceptions of friendship and positive social networks within a nursing home. *The Gerontologist, 56,* 855–867.

32 Moyle et al., p. 1446.

33 Campo, M., & Chaudhury, H. (2011). Informal social interaction among residents with dementia in special care units: Exploring the role of the physical and social environments. *Dementia, 11*, 401–423.

34 Doyle, P. J., Rubinstein, R. L., & de Medeiros, K. (2015). Generative acts of people with dementia in a long-term-care setting. *Dementia, 14*, 409–417. (p. 411)

Chapter 7

Reimagining Community

The dementia-friendly community harbors the possibility of re-imagining and re-building a society of isolated individuals in which only paid service providers provide the help needed by individuals. Understood this way, dementia-friendly communities are about inventing a new way of living with each other rather than just next to each other.

—Verena Rothe, Gabriele Kruetzner, and Reimer Gronemeyer, *Staying in Life: Paving the Way to Dementia-Friendly Communities*[1]

Friendly

Aware

Capable

Enabling

Inclusive

Positive

Supportive

These words have been used to describe community efforts to enable people to live as well as possible with a dementia. At the top of the list is "friendly," likely the most common word used in journal articles, online PDFs, books, and other media pieces about new ways of thinking about dementia and community. But different constituencies, for their own reasons, may focus on other words. One example is health-care organizations, which sometimes describe themselves as being "dementia capable" if they have intentionally developed policies, practices, and environmental designs for their facilities in light of the needs and desires of people having dementia. Because of sensitivity to professional boundaries, and to federal HIPAA[2] regulations, they would not claim to be "friendly" because that would imply relationships of mutuality and closeness deemed inappropriate for medical settings. Another example is organizations that focus on community education; for them, the word "aware" is often more important, as they emphasize their efforts to increase awareness about dementia and ways they can be supportive to people having dementia.

Although Australian dementia activist Kate Swaffer, introduced in Chapters 4 and 5, would not be surprised to see "friendly" at the top of the list above, she has been critical of facile uses of the word. She notes that people can be simultaneously friendly and patronizing.[3] Friendliness can be a smokescreen; it can hide the fact that people with dementia are treated as if they lack strengths and capabilities, as if they have nothing to contribute to the design of programs that might benefit them.[4] In a blog post commenting on Swaffer's objections, geriatrician and author G. Allen Power echoes her concerns and urges people to stop being friendly. He says that communities should focus instead on being inclusive.[5] Similarly, other authors who agree that friendliness can be superficial prefer to emphasize strengths and capabilities and urge communities to identify as being "dementia enabling and positive."

I have no objection to any of these words. They all reflect the fact that people in communities of varying types and sizes around the world are addressing the stigma and resulting isolation and exclusion of so many persons living with dementia. In fact, if this were a multiple-choice test, I think that "all of the above" would be a good answer. Even better, if our multiple-choice test were to allow an answer such as "A and B," I would opt for the words "inclusive" and "friendly." To me, those words mean that people living with a dementia (both people with the condition and their care partners) would have a say in all decisions about community efforts to create better conditions for them, and, at the same time, they would experience warm, caring, mutual relationships with fellow community members.

And yet, it is important to pause to acknowledge that the default configuration of many friendship networks is to spend time with "people like me." We need to recognize that a community where all people having dementia can live as well as possible with their progressive condition will include "people who are not like me." This is where the idea of social citizenship becomes significant.

A Social Model of Dementia

Affirming the social citizenship of persons with dementia means acting on the belief that all individuals have certain rights and, as much as possible given the nature and degree of the disability, responsibilities. We can easily imagine Grace (introduced in the last chapter) advocating for Suzy's social citizenship. However, supporting the social citizenship of all persons regardless of cognitive status does not require committing to the kind of virtuous and exemplary friendship enjoyed by Suzy and Grace. It does require that people embrace a social model of dementia, meaning that the condition is not just an issue of health to be defined in a narrow medical sense.[6] Rather, the person with dementia is understood to live in community—in relationship—with others.

Dementia is a social experience. Care is a social experience. However, the current emphasis on describing dementia mainly in terms of cognitive loss and brain changes focuses attention on individual deficits—low scores on mental tests, cerebral shrinkage, and so forth—not social relationships. Consider this quote from a book coedited by Gaynor Macdonald, whose husband has Alzheimer's disease: "Instead of starting with dementia as a cruel, feared, and vilified disease, let us start with a revaluing of vulnerability and care as intrinsic to all life."[7] By reframing it like this, Macdonald and her coauthors say that dementia becomes a social issue that "affects whole families, neighborhoods, and society at large."[8]

Relationships with people with dementia take many forms. Some affirm and support a sense of valuable selfhood and can be positive expressions of a self-fulfilling prophecy. This means that if I expect that my loved one having severe dementia can still participate in a creative-engagement activity or that she can show her love for me with a smile and a squeeze of the hand, then she will probably be more likely to live up to that expectation. Or, to use an example of someone with less severe dementia, if Grace expects that she and Suzy can have an enjoyable afternoon attending a memory café together, regardless of the fact that Suzy often repeats herself and shows other signs of her dementia, then they will be more likely to share a couple of hours of social fun. However, if Grace only sees Suzy as someone experiencing decline, loss, and terrible things happening in her brain, then when Grace encounters Suzy on a bad day, Grace might attribute her behavior to her disease, when in fact Suzy might actually be experiencing pain, hunger, loneliness, boredom, or helplessness. It is quite possible that Suzy could sense Grace's belief and respond with more withdrawal or hostility—a self-fulfilling prophecy.[9]

To view dementia in terms of decline, loss, and a diseased brain may obscure what is really bothering the person, thus leading to more behaviors that reinforce limited and negative perspectives. This spiraling accumulation of negative attitudes evoking negative behaviors that reinforce more negative attitudes can result in shaming and exclusion. Not only can shaming and exclusion be expressed interpersonally but they can also be embedded in the design of physical environments, the enactment of public policies focused solely on cost containment, and the reduction of a whole person to a health category requiring only medical care.

Observations of reductionist approaches to care with people having dementia moved Tom Kitwood to write about how "malignant social psychology" can affect mental and physical health. Some examples he offered reflect situations in which people having dementia are infantilized, intimidated, stigmatized, ignored, mocked, or ignored.[10] These social behaviors by family members or paid caregivers (many of whom may genuinely care about the individual) can hasten the self-fulfilling prophecy of decline. This is an example of what gerontologist Elaine Brody and colleagues famously called "excess disability,"[11] which refers to a person's functioning at a lower level than their disability would predict, often because care partners are focusing on the person's limitations rather than their strengths.

It is challenging enough to experience the memory loss, confusion, and emotional turmoil that come with dementia, but piling on shaming and exclusion can make matters much worse. Communities that embrace all the terms in the list at the beginning of this chapter are more likely to resist the stereotypes that produce the shaming and exclusion.

Communities in the Twenty-First Century

My family knows how much I love maps. Even today, with easily accessible digital maps, I still get much pleasure from studying folded paper maps from interstate rest stops as well as maps that appear in printed atlases. I like looking at maps of the moon and maps of the ocean floor, but my favorite maps depict places on earth where humans dwell.

Picture a typical map. On it will be roads, rivers, lakes, and perhaps an ocean. It will also include human communities, some with unusual and amusing names. These communities vary by location on the map (urban, suburban, and rural, for example) and by shading (large areas for cities; pinpoints for villages). The mapped indicators of community can tell us a lot about human life, such as how far people have to travel for food, how crowded they may feel where they live, how close they are to wonders of the natural world, and how easily they can access public transportation to go to other parts of their communities or around the world. Geographers would undoubtedly add many more items to that list. What maps cannot tell us is how people feel about their communities, whether the community itself is part of their identity, and whether they experience meaningful connections with people and places in their community.

Someone once asked me if the activities of a dementia-friendly community only occur in small towns, and my answer was no. After all, people living in cities often develop a psychological sense of community defined by their neighborhoods and the people they interact with regularly in shops, at subway stops, and in parks. Idealized images of small town, rural life still persist alongside views of big cities as hostile to creating meaningful human connections. Although there may occasionally be a kernel of truth in these stereotypes, we also know that malicious gossip can contaminate community life in small towns, and that healthy, happy relationships can form, grow, and be nurtured in big cities.

People can identify with several communities at the same time, some overlapping and others completely separate. For many years, social scientists have researched the different roles people have in their lives, and each of these roles can be enacted in different communities. In my role as mother when my children still lived at home, I connected with communities formed with other parents through school and scout organizations. One of my other roles, as a college professor in another city, did not matter when I was serving hot dogs in a school gym or squirming through a cave with Cub Scouts. During those active parenting years, in my role as professor I identified with the gerontology community consisting of people who read each other's books and journal articles and attended the same conferences. This community had no overlap with the other communities defined by my parenting roles, and vice versa.[12]

Although I could add more examples of overlap and separation of communities, one more will suffice: the virtual community. People now develop important emotional ties to online groups that meet their need for love, belongingness, and usefulness and consist of people they will never meet. This is happening throughout "dementia world" (a term popular with some online participants). Two examples of groups on Facebook include Memory People (which introduced me to memory cafés) and Purple Angel Ambassadors. On Twitter, some of the groups I follow are YoungDementia UK, Dementia Alliance International (which was founded by Kate Swaffer and colleagues), Arts4Dementia, Dementia Adventure, and Dementia Friends. Sometimes people participate in multiple online communities such that a person having dementia or a care partner might rely on several Facebook groups for information and support in coping with dementia symptoms while also participating in social-media sites for dog lovers, knitters, or gamers. There can be overlap among the dementia care-partners and the knitters, for example, but for the most part the virtual world offers membership in separate communities.

Overlap and separation can also describe brick-and-mortar communities that are dementia friendly. For example, a woman with dementia might live in a community where local businesses have been trained in how to be appropriately supportive to clients and customers having dementia. And her place of worship might have also received training in being dementia friendly and dementia inclusive. Whether she is buying bananas at a convenience store or collecting the Sunday offering, the woman feels welcomed and included. However, she might also belong to a bowling league within that community that has no patience for people who can no longer correctly keep score.

Before diving deeper into the "how to" literature of dementia-friendly and inclusive communities in the next chapter, I want to note two emerging issues in the literature: the particular challenges faced by people living with dementia in rural areas, and the growing practice of segregating people with dementia into residential care communities. Both topics deserve book-length treatment, but for now, a few pages will have to suffice.

Rural Life with Dementia

A common—and often accurate—image of rural life with dementia consists of an elderly couple living far from neighbors with very limited access to health care and services such as support groups, memory cafés, respite services, and home health care. Their children cannot find employment nearby so they relocate, sometimes far away. Internet connectivity is non-existent or painfully slow, and there is no public transportation. Financial hardships compound these challenges.[13] When one spouse or partner dies, the isolation can grow exponentially.

However, the story of rural life with dementia is not all negative. Some recent studies have indicated that there is another story we can tell, a story of neighbors caring for one another and communities supporting strong social networks.

In their research on ways people with early-stage dementia and care partners perceive dementia stigma, Sandy Burgener and her colleagues compared people living in urban Chicago and Greensboro, North Carolina, with residents of rural parts of central Illinois and Iowa. The people living in the urban areas scored higher on the level of impact they felt from dementia stigma and also the shame they felt around others due to their dementia. The authors initially thought that they would obtain opposite results because of the geographic constraints on social connectedness in rural regions. However, their data led them to suggest that in rural settings people have a stronger sense of community that "may allow for both higher levels of acceptance of someone diagnosed with dementia and the resultant changes in that person, while allowing the person diagnosed with dementia to relate to their world with more comfort."[14] With no training or official designation as "dementia friendly," these rural communities were demonstrating most of the characteristics of dementia-friendly communities.

Research conducted in rural communities of Ontario, Canada, similarly showed that people living with dementia remained connected to their social networks and that community members were ready to offer support.[15] The authors described a culture of care in which the community provided a safety net. Like so many rural communities, the ones studied in Canada experienced out-migration of young people seeking employment. Nevertheless, a strong sense of civic responsibility remained, with many of the people interviewed describing how "people look out for each other."[16] If, for example, someone appeared to be lost, neighbors would usually redirect that individual back home. In friendship networks, people seemed accepting of the changes taking place in friends having dementia. They spoke about their willingness to continue in relationship with friends even when they relocated to residential care settings. In addition, often the long-term-care staff came from the same rural region and knew the families of residents, and vice versa. However, after describing the positive aspects of a caring rural community, the authors cautioned that these connections were fragile due to increasing numbers of elders, fewer younger people, and the economic challenges of contemporary rural life. Social pressures can threaten dementia friendliness regardless of the size of the community.

Another paper about aging in a rural community reported on a study of a nursing home in a small town (population 2,800 in 1990) in Kentucky. Residents of this rural Appalachian nursing home retained the identities they had formed through living in their community for many years. They felt a strong sense of continuity with their past. This contributed to "a high level of permeability of the institution, manifest in easy and ongoing exchanges of resources, people, and information" between the nursing home and the wider community.[17] Contradicting the social stereotype that younger people do not care about elders, "community culture in this part of Appalachia involves a high level of intergenerational obligation."[18] As a result, residents regularly interacted with younger relatives, and with staff members who knew their grandchildren. In other words, numerous kinship links existed among residents, their families, and staff.

This positive view of a nursing home occupying such a significant place in a rural community should not be over-romanticized, as the authors warned in their conclusion. Moreover, given the publication date of 1996 for this paper, it would be interesting to return for a follow-up study, given contemporary concerns about the fracturing of rural communities caused by economic distress and opioid addiction. Also, the population of the nursing home today would probably be different from that of 1996, because in all likelihood there would be a higher percentage of residents having some type of dementia. (Since the 1990s, younger and healthier elders have gravitated to assisted living, leaving nursing homes with more older people with dementia.)

Residential Care Communities
Dementia Villages
Every so often a well-meaning friend excitedly sends me an article about Hogewey, a Dutch dementia village. Built in 2009, this village has attracted much positive press since it opened. In 2013 a lengthy CNN television report by Dr. Sanjay Gupta described it in glowing terms, except perhaps for the statement that residents can go "wherever they want to go except into the real world."[19] Six to eight residents live in each of several small, communal homes located on four acres, where they can shop in a supermarket (where no money is accepted), stop in to chat in a barbershop, get a cup of coffee in a small café, or just stroll along a street made to look like one in a typical small town. Staff wear street clothes and do their best to look as if they are just part of any normal village as they do things such as check people's groceries while standing at a register. Nowhere does this village look like a stereotypical nursing home with long, narrow hallways, nursing stations, and large congregate dining areas.

The idea of creating movie sets where people with dementia can live securely (for they cannot "elope" beyond the perimeter) has attracted considerable attention worldwide since Hogewey (also spelled Hogeweyk) opened. Now another village is being planned in British Columbia, Canada,[20] and one has opened in Tasmania.[21] A day center in San Diego worked with professional set designers from an opera company to create the Glenner Town Square, a faux Main Street as it might have appeared between 1953 and 1961. That specific range of time was selected because most of the participants were teenagers in those years, and psychological studies have shown the teens to be the best recalled of any life period.[22] The designers believe that the Main Street offers environmental support for reminiscence therapy.[23] Similarly, the Lantern, an assisted-living center in Ohio, offers faux front porches facing walkways bordered with fake grass, clouds painted on the ceiling of what is actually a very large warehouse-like building, different scents spritzed into the environment depending on the time of day, and recordings of bird songs played through a PA system.[24]

I can find no scientific studies of outcomes for residents of these dementia villages, but anecdotal reports from the organizations that operate them state that residents eat and sleep better, have fewer falls, take fewer medications, and overall appear to enjoy a greater quality of life compared to residents of a typical nursing home. These are all good, life-affirming outcomes, so why do these places make me so uncomfortable? Is it because I doubt that I would feel at home there, having never lived in a small village? Or, is it because at my age (71) and with my personal history and preferences, a reminiscence village would have to look more like New York City's Greenwich Village in the 1970s and not a small town in the 1950s? Can I wear my patched-up jeans and listen to Blondie and Patti Smith?

Reimagining Residential Care Communities

When my friends send me stories about dementia villages, I know they are doing so because they genuinely desire a more life-affirming approach to care. I also know that many people having dementia need 24/7 care to a degree no longer possible for loving relatives and friends, and I certainly do not want to return to a time of hospital wards and large, ugly dayrooms with blaring televisions. Memory-care communities—with and without faux accoutrements—are springing up all over the United States and in many other parts of the world as well. Many offer excellent care, although the standards of care regulated by government agencies vary widely.

Given projections of the number of persons likely to develop some type of dementia in the next 30 years, I can envision no way that even a small portion of these people will be able to live in some kind of residential care community (let alone a dementia village). Costs will be prohibitive for most individuals, especially in the US, because Medicare does not cover long-term care for chronic conditions like dementia. Unless people are very wealthy and can afford to pay privately, or they have low-enough incomes to qualify for Medicaid, the alternative will have to be intentional efforts by communities to ensure that people having dementia can live safely and well. Technology will assist to some degree, and already multiple businesses offer devices such as those that track people's movements, comfort them with robotic purring cats, monitor medication compliance, and enable communication with far-flung friends and relatives. However, it will take more than technology to reimagine community for people living with dementia.

If a person needs the kind of care that can no longer be provided in private homes, those individuals should continue to have opportunities to interact with people and places in the community. The Cycling Without Age program described in Chapter 1 is a good example of how communities can enable people having dementia to get out and about in the local environment. Besides riding around neighborhoods in a trishaw, long-term care residents can be invited to local cultural events. Yes, many use wheelchairs and walkers, but they can be accommodated by specially equipped vans to enable people to participate in community life. This will require changes in how staff are trained and compensated, for they would need to accompany residents, unless families or community volunteers could do this.

Some residential-care settings invite the community inside their walls by collaborating with nearby schools. Also, some incorporate day-care centers for very young children on their campuses. An innovative organization in Kentucky sponsors summer day-camps for their staff's children. Residents of these care communities have regular opportunities to interact meaningfully with the children, and the children learn about aging and dementia from residents, staff, and teachers.

A review of the literature on intergenerational programs involving people with dementia noted mostly positive outcomes both for the children and the elders. The articles studied by the authors described a wide variety of activities, such as narrative storytelling, singing, gardening, baking, and nature walks. The particular activity or art form did not appear to matter as much as the opportunities afforded for relationship building. The studies summarized in this paper showed that the people with dementia appreciated having a meaningful social role, increased self-confidence, and greater social engagement.[25]

In Japan, Mizuhashi House, a group home for people having dementia located near several schools, developed a unique program for residents to act as patrol guards for the children. Residents even had homemade uniforms to wear when standing at a watch station observing the children going to and from school. By having adults on duty—in this case, elders with dementia—students, parents, and school staff reported that they experienced a greater sense of safety. One unexpected positive outcome was that residents were so dedicated to performing their duties that they got much more outdoor exercise in the winter months.[26]

Bringing memory-care residents to the community and bringing the community to residents is one way to reimagine community. Doing so would address one of my pet peeves in the dementia literature: the statement that 70 percent of people having dementia live in the community. This gets repeated in many documents, from official government reports on unpaid caregiving to pleas for financial support from the Alzheimer's Association. But what does it really mean? It implies that when you relocate to some form of long-term care you are no longer considered part of your community. So where do you live? On Mars?

Activists like Kate Swaffer talk about the "ghetto-ization" of people with dementia living in places—even the fancy ones—where they have no access to the world beyond the walls of the building or perhaps its gardens. Anne Basting has expressed concern about the creation of a "parallel universe for people with dementia."[27] For German theologian and sociologist Reimer Gronemeyer, the story of Tithonos from Greek mythology supplies an image of long-term care residences cut off from their communities: he calls them Tithonos cages.

Tithonos was the prince of Troy. His lover, Eos (the goddess of dawn), asked Zeus to make him immortal. Unfortunately, she forgot to ask that he remain forever young. When he became disabled in multiple ways by age and shrank to the size of a cicada, Eos locked him in a cage. Gronemeyer applied the story to contemporary life like this:

> ...the number of Tithonos cages is rather likely to grow. In them, we can be looked after, but participating in life we do not. It is, however, possible to imagine that nursing homes do not see themselves as custodial institutions but rather open their doors to a surrounding community that has itself discovered that it might be interested in those who have been shunted off or are in need of care.[28]

Reimagining community in light of increasing numbers of persons having dementia will require changes in attitudes, language, policies, and practices. One way to open the doors of the Tithonos cages would be to view nursing homes and other forms of residential care not merely as health-care providers but as community resources offering arts, cultural, and intergenerational experiences for residents, staff, families, and community members.

Today, various types of residential care communities seem to pop up like mushrooms in our cities, towns, and villages. People live alongside them, barely paying attention to what goes on inside their walls. When I give lectures about this situation, I often show a photograph of an ancient British castle surrounded by a moat. Whether it is a building designated for assisted living, skilled nursing care, or memory care, or it is a campus that includes all of these plus so-called "independent living," the invisible moat can seem impregnable to all but staff and family members.

If communities are truly going to be dementia friendly and inclusive (along with all the other descriptors listed at the beginning of this chapter), then they need to educate their citizens to view people with dementia and other expressions of frailty as having something valuable to contribute to community life. By doing so, they could do what was suggested in the epigraph that began this chapter: help us invent new ways of living with each other. This could produce new ways of thinking about disabilities of all kinds, thinking undergirded by commitments to uphold human rights for everyone. After all, if we commit to ending prejudice and discrimination against persons with dementia, then—given their diversity not only in diagnosis and place on the dementia-progression spectrum but also in culture, language, religion, sexuality, gender identity, and skin color—we might also hope that commitment would generalize to honoring human rights for all persons.

Endnotes

1   Rothe, V., Kruetzner, G., & Gronemeyer, R. (2017). *Staying in life: Paving the way to dementia-friendly communities*. Bielefeld, Germany: Transcript-Verlag. Reprinted by permission of Transcript Verlag.

2   In the US, HIPAA stands for the Health Insurance Portability and Accountability Act, signed by President Clinton in 1996. It applies to people working in health-care organizations ranging from nursing homes to hospitals as well as health-insurance providers. HIPAA regulations prevent them from sharing information about residents/patients without written permission. Increasingly, the focus is on data breaches in which computer records are accessed illegally.

3   This idea that friendships can have toxic elements may have led the AARP to revise its efforts to promote age-friendly cities and instead to encourage the creation of livable communities. Note also the change from "cities" to "communities." See: www.aarp.org/livable-communities

4   Rahman, S., & Swaffer, K. (2018). Assets-based approaches and dementia-friendly communities. *Dementia, 17*, 131–137.

5   Power, G. A. (2014, December 2). *Can we stop being "dementia-friendly"?* [Blog post]. Changing Aging. Accessed on 7/22/19 at https://changingaging.org/dementia/can-we-stop-being-dementia-friendly

6   Henwood, C., & Downs, M. (2014). Dementia-friendly communities. In M. Downs & B. Bowers (Eds.), *Excellence in dementia care: Research into practice* (2nd ed., pp. 20–35). Maidenhead, UK: Open University Press.

7   Macdonald, G., Mears, J., & Naderbagi, A. (2019). Reframing dementia: The social imperative. In G. Macdonald & J. Mears (Eds.), *Dementia as social experience: Valuing life and care* (pp. 1–19). New York, NY: Routledge. (p. 1)

8   Macdonald et al., p. 2.

9   Social psychologists refer to this as the fundamental attribution error. That means that people attribute their own behavior to external causes (I honked my car horn at that person because he was too slow to move when the light changed) but they attribute other people's behavior to internal causes (that driver who honked at me is an angry, bad person).

10 Kitwood, T. (1997). *Dementia reconsidered: The person comes first*. Philadelphia, PA: Open University Press. (pp. 45–53)
See also: Sabat, S. R. (2001). *The experience of Alzheimer's disease: Life through a tangled veil*. Malden, MA: Blackwell Publishers.

11 Brody, E. M., Kelban, M. H., Lawton, M. P., & Silverman, H. A. (1971). Excess disabilities of mentally impaired aged: Impact of individualized treatment. *The Gerontologist, 11*(2, Pt. 1), 124–133.

12 The issue of overlapping roles and identities is sometimes presented as evidence of intersectionality, a term used in academic circles to describe the interconnection of social identities such as race, gender, class, and sexuality. Intersectionality was first emphasized by black feminists. For a review of intersectionality theory and social practice, see: Oleksy, E. H. (2011). Intersectionality at the cross-roads. *Women's Studies International Forum, 34*, 263–270.

13 Easter Seals Disability Services and the National Alliance for Caregiving conducted a study of rural caregiving of all types, including care for children with disabilities, disabled veterans (almost 25 percent of all veterans live in rural areas), and people who sustained injuries on their farm or ranch. See: Hunt, G., Johnson, J., Maus, C., & Brugger, M. (2006). *Caregiving in rural America*. Washington, DC: Easter Seals and The National Alliance for Caregiving. Accessed on 7/22/19 at www.caregiving.org/wp-content/uploads/2014/01/Easter-Seals_NAC_Caregiving_in_Rural.pdf

14 Burgener, S. C., Buckwalter, K., Perkhounkova, Y., Liu, M. F., Riley, R., Einhorn, C. J., et al. (2015). Perceived stigma in persons with early-stage dementia: Longitudinal findings: Part 1. *Dementia, 14*, 589–608. (p. 603)

15 Wiersma & Denton, (2016). From social network to safety net: Dementia-friendly communities in rural northern Ontario. *Dementia, 15*(1), 51–68.

16 Wiersma & Denton, p. 58.

17 Rowles, G. D., Concotelli, J. A., & High, D. M. (1996). Community integration of a rural nursing home. *Journal of Applied Gerontology, 15*, 188–201. (p. 189)

18 Rowles et al., p. 194.

19 www.youtube.com/watch?v=LwiOBlyWpko

20 https://bc.ctvnews.ca/canada-s-first-dementia-village-set-to-open-its-doors-1.4441535

21 www.agedcareguide.com.au/talking-aged-care/tasmania-to-be-home-to-australias-first-dementia-village?sfns=mo

22 Psychologists call this the "reminiscence bump." People over 40 have the most autobiographical memories from adolescence and early adulthood. See this review of current literature on the reminiscence bump: Koppel, J., & Rubin, D. C. (2016). Recent advances in understanding the reminiscence bump: The importance of cues in guiding recall from autobiographical memory. *Current Directions in Psychological Science, 25*, 135–140.

23 https://glenner.org/town-square/town-square-faq

24 Pennell, J. (2016, August 31). This home for people with Alzheimer's is going viral for its resort-like design. *TODAY*. Accessed on 7/23/19 at www.today.com/home/lantern-assisted-living-t102373

25 Galbraith, B., Larkin, H., Moorhouse, A., & Oomen, T. (2015). Intergenerational programs for persons with dementia: A scoping review. *Journal of Gerontological Social Work, 58*, 357–378.

26 Kellehear, A. (2009). Dementia and dying: The need for a systematic policy approach. *Critical Social Policy, 29*, 146–157.

27 Peters, K. R., & Katz, S. (2015). Interview with Dr. Anne Davis Basting, 21 May 2013. *Dementia, 14*(3), 328–334. (p. 331)
28 Gronemeyer, R. (2017). The dementia-friendly community: A daring venture. In V. Rothe, G. Kreutzner, & R. Gronemeyer (Eds.), *Staying in life: Paving the way to dementia-friendly communities* (pp. 17–41). Bielefeld, Germany: Transcript-Verlag. (p. 36)

Chapter 8

Creating Dementia-Friendly and Inclusive Communities

In 2005, the World Health Organization (WHO) launched a program to promote age-friendly cities based on input from 33 cities in 22 countries.[1] An extensive checklist of features of these cities described age-friendly ideals for outdoor spaces and buildings, transportation, housing, social participation, respect and social inclusion, civic participation and employment, communication and information, and community and health services. Age-friendly cities were envisioned as places that would

- include and welcome people of all ages and backgrounds

- support meaningful social interaction

- encourage health in body, mind, and spirit

- be accessible

- foster interdependence among neighbors and across generations

- promote various forms of community engagement.[2]

But wait! What happens when an elder living in one of these age-friendly cities develops dementia? In 2011, the UK organization Innovations in Dementia noted that the WHO document failed to recognize that a high percentage of elders in age-friendly cities would develop dementia. This group embraced a rights-based approach to dementia described in Chapter 5, arguing that dementia should not interfere with the right to a good life in one's community.

Founded as an advocacy group in 2007, Innovations in Dementia described characteristics of what it called dementia-capable communities.[3] Their work is significant because it resulted from online surveys as well as telephone and face-to-face interviews with people having dementia, supporters of people with dementia (mostly family members), and people who worked or volunteered with people having dementia. The group spoke to people in memory cafés, at a drop-in center, and in public gathering spaces, including a library, coffee shop, gym, and even a pub. These were located in rural, urban, and suburban regions.

The central question for everyone interviewed was "Which aspects of a community make it a good place to live for people with dementia?"[4] The report contains many quotes from participants who described not only what made their communities good places but also what made their communities difficult to live in. They described things they had stopped doing since developing dementia and told what they wished they could still do if certain barriers were removed.

The refrain heard repeatedly in this work was that people wanted to be able to continue to do the things they had always enjoyed, but they were encountering many obstacles to that goal in their communities. One person from the rural area stated this succinctly by saying that it is important to be "somewhere you can see life going on and be part of it."[5]

Of the many quotes I could cite from this document, which contains many insightful quotes from people having dementia reflecting on things that help or prevent them from living well in their communities, the following statement particularly captured my attention and made me realize how an ordinary action I love and take for granted—going to the library—can be so challenging for someone with dementia:

> I have stopped using the library because they have introduced self-checkout and I'm worried what will happen if I get it wrong—or if I can't keep track of when my books are meant to be returned. They don't stamp it in the front of the book like they used to, and I'd need someone to help with that.[6]

This library patron sounds like many people who do not want to bother someone else by asking for assistance. Perhaps they also feel reluctant because they sense the stigma associated with their condition. However, a librarian trained to be alert to a patron's need for assistance without reinforcing the stigma could helpfully offer to check out the book and insert a note saying when it is due back at the library. And would it be too burdensome for the librarian to offer to call the person to say the book is due? Libraries today send emails about overdue books, but how does that help people who do not use email?

These questions may seem inconsequential in light of the loud and constant messages about increasing numbers of persons having a brain disease producing some type of dementia, the lack of medical fixes, and the resulting burden to societies. And yet, addressing these types of issues related to everyday life can help people living with dementia feel supported and included in their communities. The dementia-friendly community movement now springing up in many parts of the world seeks to articulate ways to offer this support and inclusion.

Enter "dementia-friendly community" into any internet search engine and pages of documents pop up. Many of them are in the form of "toolkits" that list characteristics of such communities and suggestions about strategies to achieve them. One of the first appeared in 2013; it was created by the Alzheimer's Society in the United Kingdom. This document cited the following 10 key components of dementia-friendly communities. They should

- involve people with dementia

- challenge dementia stigma and build understanding about dementia

- ensure that community activities are accessible

- acknowledge the potential of people having dementia

- make early diagnosis available to all

- offer practical support [such as checking out library books] for ongoing engagement with community life

- provide community-based solutions based on what communities determine is needed

- be certain that travel options are reliable and consistent

- determine that environments are easy to navigate

- have businesses and services that are respectful and responsible.[7]

The Alzheimer's Society report containing this list aligned with Prime Minister David Cameron's challenge on dementia issued in 2012. This means that in the UK, creation of dementia-friendly communities was a national policy initiative from the beginning. Its goals were to improve health and social care for people having dementia, encourage the development of dementia-friendly communities, and support research on dementia. Earlier, in 2009, the UK's Department of Health published the National Dementia Strategy, a five-year plan to benefit people with dementia, care partners, health and social-services professionals, and anyone else affected by dementia. The intent was to make it possible for the policy directing the creation of dementia-friendly communities to be carried out locally.[8]

One of the notable characteristics of the UK's National Dementia Strategy is its affirmation that people having dementia are citizens. It does not begin with the assumption that these are helpless individuals in need of care because they have a brain disease. Rather, they are friends, neighbors, and family members who have been a part of their communities for a long time. The strategy communicated a public-health approach that acknowledges the need for various types of direct services for people living with dementia, but it situated those services within an approach that relies upon community engagement.[9]

Communities throughout the UK took various approaches to recruiting stakeholders and creating networks that could join together to do the work of achieving the goals articulated by the Alzheimer's Society and the UK's National Dementia Strategy. This was often easier said than done, as documented in a study of challenges communities face in doing this work. For example, stakeholders may initially respond with enthusiasm, but that can wane as the hard work of creating and sustaining networks moves forward. Although the idea of including persons having dementia in these efforts is a kind of "gold standard" for this work, actually making that happen can be difficult, given the everyday challenges they face.[10]

In the United States, the first fully realized dementia-friendly community effort began in Minnesota. There the ACT on Alzheimer's organization developed a free online toolkit to guide communities in gathering stakeholders, assessing needs and resources, determining priorities for action, and creating an action plan. ACT on Alzheimer's realized that communities would differ in their priorities and their resources for developing and carrying out their plans. The organization worked with many Minnesota communities, ranging from big cities such as St. Paul to small towns in the northern part of the state called the Iron Range. Based on its success distributing the toolkit and coaching community groups in its use, in 2015 ACT on Alzheimer's morphed into a national organization called Dementia Friendly America. Its website defines a dementia-friendly community as "a village, town, city, or county that is informed; is safe and respectful of individuals with the disease, their families and caregivers; and provides supportive options that foster quality of life."[11]

Like many of the other organizations one can access with an internet search for "dementia-friendly communities," Dementia Friendly America urges interested persons to begin by learning what people living with dementia want from their communities. Then, together, they need to identify a vision, goals, and a timeline for achieving their goals, along with a way to support them financially. Community partners should be identified, and coalitions and partnerships need to be built with various interested persons and organizations. The list of possible activities to nurture dementia friendliness is lengthy, including but not limited to

- educating people of all ages about dementia

- training customer-facing employees of businesses and organizations to respond helpfully and respectfully to persons having dementia

- making environmental alterations for easier way-finding

- developing memory cafés and other activities for people with dementia to share with care partners

- identifying needed changes in policies and practices in health-care organizations.

In addition to offering a structured approach for communities to develop dementia-friendly initiatives, Dementia Friendly America also coordinates the Dementia Friends program in the US.[12] The Alzheimer's Society in the UK began this program and now licenses organizations worldwide to provide structured, brief training to citizens in how to think, act, and talk about dementia. People of all ages are invited to be trained as a Dementia Friend and then to act on what they have learned when connecting with people having dementia. In the US, many state dementia networks are signing on to this program. For example, Minnesota set and achieved a goal of training 10,000 Dementia Friends in 2018.

In their state-of-the-science review of research on dementia-friendly initiatives, Catherine Hebert and Kezia Scales identify 241 relevant journal articles, with 80 percent of them appearing after 2011 and most having been published in Europe or the UK. After reviewing this literature, they conclude that it represents "a transformative change in society's view of living with dementia."[13]

This transformative change is occurring worldwide. In a paper on dementia-friendly communities, Cathy Henwood and Murna Downs give examples from Germany, Japan, Belgium, and the UK. They advocate for the "Four Cornerstones Model" developed by the Joseph Rowntree Foundation in the UK. It defines the cornerstones of a dementia-friendly community as place, people, resources, and networks. This model was also employed by the Alzheimer Europe organization in its 2015 report on dementia-friendly communities in 26 European Union member states (including the UK at the time) and five non-EU member states.[14] It is also the model used to develop Fox Valley Memory Project (FVMP), the dementia-friendly community effort with which I am most familiar because I helped to create the organization.[15] When several colleagues and I began working on FVMP in 2011, we had no idea that we were building upon those four cornerstones! Nevertheless, we defined a place, invited people (including those living with dementia) to join us in forming the organization, obtained resources from local philanthropic organizations and a few initial donors, and networked with organizations including the local chapter of the Alzheimer's Association, Wisconsin's Department of Health Services, the regional Aging and Disability Resource Center, a family-medicine residency clinic, and Goodwill Industries.

Starting with Memory Cafés: A Case Example from Fox Valley Memory Project

Often, a community eases its way into becoming dementia friendly and inclusive by establishing a memory café. Just as there are many toolkits available online that offer concrete recommendations for launching dementia-friendly community efforts, so, too, are there many that describe how to start and sustain memory cafés. I have included an appendix with a list of these websites and brief descriptions of their content.

Memory cafés (occasionally called Alzheimer's cafés) welcome people living with dementia, along with their family care-partners and friends, to enjoy about two hours of socializing in an accessible, comfortable, and welcoming space with no concerns about dementia stigma. Usually there is some kind of program, but sometimes people attending a café just want to interact informally with other participants. When organizers plan entertainment, they try to make it interactive rather than passive. For example, at a recent memory café where my husband, John, and I volunteer, a string quartet consisting of members of our local symphony played for about 45 minutes while encouraging participants to sing, dance in their chairs, wave colorful scarves, and wear hats reflecting the day's theme of cowboy music.

Memory cafés can be located in actual cafés, but most occur in settings such as libraries, community centers, nature centers, churches, and other spaces with accessible parking or public transportation. No matter the location, the most important theme in the literature on memory cafés is inclusive hospitality. Although some memory cafés advertise being for people in the early stage of dementia, I have never heard of people being refused entry because their dementia has progressed. In fact, we have some family members who pick up their loved ones at residential care communities and bring them to memory cafés. This means that their dementia has progressed to the point that they can no longer live independently or with a loved one but they still enjoy attending familiar group activities designed to make them feel welcome and comfortable.

The efforts of care partners to accompany loved ones from care communities illustrate an important point: memory cafés are just as much for the care partners as they are for the people living with dementia. Care partners become friends with other participants. Because hospitality is woven into everything that happens at the café, care partners do not have to worry about their loved ones' behavior or what they say or do not say. We promote the idea that people leave their dementia diagnosis at the door when they enter a memory café. In fact, we have had several visitors comment that they cannot tell who has dementia and who does not.

Memory café hospitality is evident from the moment people arrive and are greeted by volunteers who give them nametags and invite them to relax and get comfortable in the room. The nametags are important, so we take care in how we make them. Each nametag consists of a plastic sleeve over a three-by-four-inch paper label that has the person's name printed in bold, large letters (size 48 font) along with FVMP's logo. We attach a chain to the top corners to make them easy to wear and to prevent the nametags from flipping over to their blank sides (as so easily happens with nametags attached to lanyards). Receiving a nametag upon entering the café and then returning it to a volunteer when the café time ends becomes a kind of ritual. Everyone gets a nametag, including all guests and volunteers. This simple gesture contributes to the welcoming feeling of group cohesiveness. This is important, especially for people who have become socially isolated due to their own or their partner's dementia symptoms.

During or after the café's main activity, volunteers offer people coffee or tea and some kind of treat. Nothing needs to be fancy or expensive, and everything should reflect the preferences of the group. Occasionally we have activities that involve learning about food, in which case we offer related treats. For example, because FVMP is a Wisconsin program, we once invited the owner of a local dairy to talk to the group. This dairy has operated in our community since 1913 so was quite familiar to most memory café participants. After hearing about the history of the company and passing around old photos and relics of dairy operations, we all enjoyed sampling their chocolate milk and regular milk—with, of course, a side of cookies.

Developing a memory café is often a bottom-up process, with a few interested persons hearing about the cafés and then figuring out how to begin offering them. Dementia-friendly community programs and policies then sometimes follow, as people consider other ways to make their communities more welcoming and supportive of those living with dementia. This is how FVMP began. Alternatively, dementia-friendly community efforts can result from a top-down process in which national, state, or regional governments or nonprofits determine that changes are needed to ensure good life quality for people having dementia. Partnerships among organizations serving older adults, including those with dementia, are formed, and priorities for necessary changes are determined. Often the first priority is to establish one or more memory cafés.

Regardless of how the dementia-friendly (and, one hopes, inclusive) community effort begins, it is usually connected in some way to one or more local memory cafés. Sometimes, as in the case of FVMP, the same organization oversees the memory cafés as well as other dementia-friendly efforts, such as educational programs, the training of businesses to respond helpfully to people living with dementia, and the persuasion of local governments to address complex but essential issues like housing and transportation. The success of a memory café can prompt a call for more community engagement for people living with dementia and more programs and services that meet their changing needs.

The Origins of Fox Valley Memory Project

But what are the nuts and bolts involved in starting a memory café? And how might a café grow into a wider dementia-friendly and inclusive community? At this point, I would like to offer a deeper look at the genesis of such a community, one that I know intimately—FVMP. I hope that its story and continued success, however imperfect, might offer inspiration for other communities. Although I will begin by describing my own and my husband's involvement, FVMP has thrived due to the hard work and collaboration of many individuals and organizations.

In 2007, my university granted me a sabbatical to study how dementia affected people's relationships with their friends and their wider communities. Over 40 years of studying, researching, and teaching about psychology had focused my attention on individuals, most of them research subjects or therapy clients. I had never learned to think about the dynamic interaction of individuals with their communities. I realized that I had failed to consider the role of decisions in larger systems (such as local governments and health-care organizations) that affected people's attempts to live as well as possible with dementia in their communities.

This thinking about community formed a major theme in a book John and I wrote about dementia and friendship.[16] John had spent his career as a pastor of large Congregational churches, so he knew a lot about the blessings and curses of community life. My sabbatical research had revealed the dearth of material on friends journeying together through the progressive changes of dementia. As John describes it, our book was more theoretical than practical, and when we finished writing it, we looked at each other and asked, "Now what?" We wondered how we could help people continue to enjoy and value their friendships even when the person with dementia no longer recalled the story of the friendship.

About that time, I stumbled across the Facebook group called "Memory People." Someone posted a statement about memory cafés in England. A brief Google search landed me on a page showing memory cafés all over England and giving contact information for the facilitators. Interestingly, I learned that many had been started by local Rotary Clubs through an organization called RePOD (Rotarians Easing Problems of Dementia). John had been a Rotarian since the mid-1970s, so this seemed like a great connection for us.

Thus began the era of what John called our "dementia tourism." I wrote emails to some of the people listed on the memory café website, and soon we had invitations not only to visit the cafés but also to stay at people's homes and attend dinners they organized for memory café volunteers. With this hospitality generously offered to us, we began planning our trip. In the summer of 2011, we flew to Manchester, England, rented a car, and drove 860 miles. We saw no British tourist attractions, but we did spend time in a lot of church basements, senior centers, and housing for elders where cafés were held. It was a marvelous experience (except for my terror on the road when John drifted to the left and came too close to stone walls and other barriers), and we are still in touch with several of the people who introduced us to memory cafés. That experience not only taught us about the core value of hospitality in memory cafés but also demonstrated the need to visit them in order to begin to grasp how they operate.

All through 2011 I had been meeting with three people in my region of northeast Wisconsin to develop a plan for serving people who were living with dementia, regardless of the dementia type or the progression of their dementia. In keeping with the Four Cornerstones Model (which, at the time, we did not know we were using), we had to determine the place where our work would be located. We were thinking big, largely inspired by the great need we had all witnessed among people experiencing loneliness, boredom, and helplessness resulting from dementia symptoms that had reduced the size of their social worlds. Should we try to serve the whole nation, the state, or our local region? We decided on the latter with the goal of developing best practices that could be shared with others. Our service area footprint matched the service area of our local community foundation, the "resource" cornerstone in the model.

We submitted successful planning grant proposals to the community foundation and another philanthropic organization and used that funding to hold a community breakfast where a large group of curious, interested people ate scrambled eggs and toast before listening to brief presentations. The term "dementia-inclusive community" had not yet become widely used, but that is what we were trying to model by inviting people living with dementia along with care partners and local thought leaders. After breakfast, they participated together in a three-hour think tank to identify strengths and weaknesses in the way our community responded to people with dementia. Then, early in 2012, we gathered and organized ideas generated at the think tank and wrote multi-year major grant applications.

Our grants were partially funded, giving us enough money to hire a part-time director and to introduce FVMP to our community. November 2012 marked the opening of our first memory café.

We now have 10 every month, meeting in eight different locations in a region encompassing an entire county and parts of three adjacent counties. Although FVMP now offers much more than memory cafés, they were our first way of demonstrating that people living with memory loss and other challenges of dementia could continue to enjoy life in our community. The cafés provide plenty of pleasure—but even more important, they offer people meaningful connections with one another. This can be readily observed on FVMP's Facebook page where we frequently post photos of people enjoying the memory cafés and other activities. Everyone whose photo appears on the Facebook page has given permission to be photographed, and we are finding that they, along with their children, grandchildren, and friends, enjoy seeing this evidence of the pleasure and social connectedness offered by FVMP programs.

John and I began facilitating FVMP's first memory café in 2012 in an actual café located in a repurposed paper mill alongside the Fox River in Appleton, Wisconsin. We met in a private room of the café that looked out onto the river through enormous old windows. We often watched eagles and white pelicans soaring over the rapid current. Reflecting their mission of serving the community, the generous owners of the café did not charge us for the space and provided coffee and treats at no charge. Our responsibilities as facilitators required John and me to plan the programs, invite guest artists or other types of presenters, keep track of who attended, and model hospitality.

After facilitating the café for six years, John and I stepped down to allow someone else to take on that role, and we became volunteers at another monthly FVMP café. We continue to volunteer at that second café, which is also located in a repurposed paper mill, on the same river a few miles north of the original café. This one is in a library—one of four libraries in our region offering memory cafés sponsored by FVMP—and this is the place where we met Grace and Suzy who were introduced in Chapter 6. Other regular participants in that café include married couples, sons and daughters who bring a parent, and occasionally a paid home caregiver accompanying a client.

From FVMP's start in 2012, we have always begun the cafés with what we call our "Hello song." With participants ranging in number from 10 to 30, John accompanies the group on his ukulele, and we go around the room naming each individual in the room, including guests and volunteers: "Hello, Kathy, how do you do? We're glad to say hello to you." Everyone waves or somehow gestures to the group when their name is sung. This small ritual is important because it gives structure to the beginning of our café time together. If anyone has a birthday that month, we sing "Happy Birthday." We then move on to announcements about upcoming FVMP services and activities. These include quarterly all-day bus trips, our chorus, monthly social meet-ups in restaurants, support groups, memory assessment at two local clinics that work closely with FVMP, and twice-weekly Mindworks brain-training activities for people living with dementia.

At FVMP we are proud of what we have accomplished, but we are acutely aware that more work remains to be done. We are still not reaching our rural communities; most of our memory cafés are clustered in cities. We know that we have more work to do to include culturally and linguistically diverse persons living with dementia. Despite holding a think tank for local human resources professionals a few years ago, we have also not made much progress in finding ways for people with younger-onset dementia to remain employed or to find meaningful volunteer work. We have partnered with a number of long-term-care communities in order to include their residents in FVMP programs, but that can be challenging because of turnover in facility staff. Nevertheless, at least annually, we hold a public event for the wider community featuring some type of arts program (described in more detail in Chapter 9) that includes residents of care communities.

Issues Needing Further Discussion

Looking beyond the example of FVMP, it is remarkable how quickly the commitment to making communities dementia friendly has grown since 2011 when Innovations in Dementia published its interviews about what people with dementia wanted and needed to make their lives work better in their rural villages, small towns, and big cities. It is also humbling to think about what else needs to be done. For example, the Dementia Friends program could benefit people living in residential care settings. There is a growing literature on bullying behaviors in residential care, often perpetrated by elders with no signs of dementia who ignore, actively exclude, or insult persons having dementia. Several newspaper articles about "mean girls" in retirement communities have poignantly described the feelings of residents who have been the targets of this unfriendly behavior.[17] Interventions have been designed to address organizational practices that may create an environment conducive to bullying. Programs aimed at helping residents stop their bullying behavior are also available, along with programs that empower residents targeted by bullies.[18]

This problem of bullying is just one of many issues that need to be addressed as the dementia-friendly and inclusive community movement matures. Creating dementia-friendly communities requires hard work by people operating at many levels of engagement with people living with dementia. As noted by Suzanne Cahill in her 2018 book on dementia and human rights, a risk exists that this movement will become all things to all people, in a negative sense:

> ...to the politician, a vote catcher; to the retailer, a new consumer group; to the service provider, a reduced caseload; and to the individual, the prospects of being labeled and having all their behavior seen only through the dementia. Of real concern is the fact that governments and policy makers may consider dementia-friendly communities low-cost solutions to the heightening challenge that dementia poses.[19]

There is also the risk that significant but difficult issues will be ignored. One risk results from the emphasis on early diagnosis that appears in nearly all documents describing dementia-friendly communities. If a dementia diagnosis comes before people are ready to retire, not only may they lose their income, and possibly their health insurance (if it is provided by their employer), but they may also lose a significant source of their meaning and purpose as an independent adult.[20] Interviews with individuals who lost their jobs due to having dementia have revealed a lack of understanding by employers, trauma for the person, and financial distress for the family. At home, out of a job, individuals felt no longer useful to other people and their communities. Often socially isolated because others in their age cohort were still working full time, some slipped into depression, which can exacerbate dementia-related cognitive problems.[21]

A related issue concerns employed dementia care-partners. Many report that their work is disrupted because of caregiving responsibilities. They use their vacation time to provide care, thus depriving themselves of opportunities to reduce stress. Taking a loved one to doctors' appointments, attending to a toileting accident just before leaving for work, or countless other interruptions in a day can force a person to be absent from work. Care partners may refuse promotions that bring more responsibility and time commitments that would interfere with their caregiving commitments. Many are forced to retire early, which results in additional financial challenges.[22]

In the US, the issue of organizational responses to employees showing signs of dementia, or to people caring for a loved one, is sometimes called the dangerous "third rail"[23] of human-resources policies and practices. Many organizations have not considered how they might provide accommodations for employees showing signs of dementia or for care partners, even though, anecdotally, they may know about employees whose work is affected by changes in cognitive functions or caregiving responsibilities. This represents a complex challenge for employers, because the expression of dementia symptoms could have tragic consequences for employees, coworkers, customers, and the public in jobs ranging from accountants managing other people's money to public-safety officers carrying guns.[24] However, if a community is truly going to commit to being dementia friendly and inclusive, then community leaders need to begin to address these workplace issues.[25]

Creating communities that welcome, include, and support people with all types of dementia, and at all levels of dementia, along with their care partners, will involve more than good-hearted, well-meaning volunteers offering a memory café in a church basement once a month. There will have to be involvement from local, state, and national government, and some of the necessary changes in policies and practices will require increased funding.

How might this money be spent? The list of possibilities is enormous because the needs are many, but I will mention two resources that can improve well-being for people with dementia and care partners: respite programs and adult day services. An example of the former could be a church that trains volunteers to lead creative-engagement programs several hours each month for people with dementia. Those few hours could make a big difference for care partners who feel as if they never have sufficient time to do things such as get their hair cut, have coffee with a friend, or even take a nap. Sometimes, county offices on aging have funds available to pay trained community members to go to people's homes to spend time with the person with dementia, thus giving respite to the care partner. People trained as Dementia Friends could also do this.

Adult day services usually provide at least eight hours of creatively designed social programming each weekday in safe, engaging environments under the leadership of well-trained people committed to respecting the personhood of all clients. These programs enable care partners to remain employed or to continue important roles such as caring for grandchildren. Adult day services also help to combat the loneliness, boredom, and helplessness experienced by so many people having dementia. However, these programs are expensive to operate, and if all the costs must be borne by participants' families, then many people will be excluded. Thus, in most communities, there needs to be some kind of public support.

The issue of raising taxes is another political "third rail" in the US and other countries. In line with citizens not wanting tax increases, and governments trying to reduce spending, we have the situation in the US of long-term-care services (both residential and in-home) increasingly being delivered by for-profit organizations. This change has been sold as a way to reduce the spending of public funds for these services, but there is actually little evidence that it works. Larry Polivka and Baozhen Luo recently offered an important analysis of this situation in the US:

> The loss of community-based LTC [long-term-care] services to outside corporate interests reduces communities' investment in the lives of their older residents and their families, and it weakens communities. The erosion of a community's sense of moral responsibility for its members, especially vulnerable members like the frail elderly, undermines any sense of collective efficacy or the sense that the community has a critical role to play in addressing policy changes like LTC.[26]

In addition to the third rails of human-resource issues and government funding for various forms of long-term care and respite services, there are other challenging issues that seldom appear in documents about how to create dementia-friendly communities. Another third rail topic no one wants to address is death. For example, after relating the story of Tithonos described in the previous chapter, Gronemeyer immediately presented readers with the troubling issue of assisted dying. As genetic tests for possible dementia risk become more widely available, this is a topic of whispered, worried discussion among more people. Recently, I thought I was having a fairly casual conversation with an acquaintance about writing this book and being motivated in part by increasing numbers of persons having dementia. She responded by sharing her worry that more people would choose to die by suicide rather than face life with a progression of dementia symptoms. This is a topic being debated by ethicists. An early example comes from the work of Stephen Post, the scholar who coined the term "hypercognitive society" to describe why people living with dementia often feel excluded from their social worlds when they can no longer meet expectations for vast memory abilities and highly organized thinking.[27] In Post's opinion, assisted suicide represents a society's refusal to care for its weakest members and is a sign of moral collapse.

In addition to ethicists, ordinary people also debate the issue of assisted suicide for people with dementia, especially after publicity of the suicides of well-known persons. For example, when the psychologist Sandra Bem was diagnosed with Alzheimer's dementia, she decided she wanted to take her own life before the disease progressed to a point where she no longer could exercise agency in ending her life. She also wanted her choice and the method she used to be made known in her obituary. An article about her decision and how she carried it out appeared in the *New York Times Magazine* and generated considerable debate.[28]

A related issue concerns the way people with dementia receive care at the end of their lives. The medicalized approach to care, combined with professional dominance over decision-making for people with dementia and their families, has produced a situation in which "the social and spiritual approaches to care are simply omitted."[29] Dementia-friendly communities need to acknowledge that dementia is a terminal condition, but that most people, whether living at home or in residential care, continue to want to interact with the wider community as long as possible. This means that there is a role for dementia-friendly training to engage people with dementia and their families in conversations about their end-of-life wishes and to encourage completion of end-of-life care-planning documents. Dementia-friendly community leaders could also work with hospice organizations to ensure that volunteers and paid staff understand how to communicate meaningfully with an individual with dementia who may no longer be able to speak but who can be comforted with gentle touch, calming scents, and soothing music.[30]

There are many other important issues seldom addressed in the literature on dementia-friendly communities. In her new book *Dementia Reimagined*, bioethicist and physician Tia Powell devotes a whole chapter to three of these: sex, driving, and money.[31] These activities of ordinary adult life raise ethical challenges for people who care about individuals living with dementia. How can families and professionals determine when an individual's right to autonomy jeopardizes safety of the person and possibly others because of the progress of that person's dementia symptoms? The answer to this question will vary according to circumstances and individual differences, but it is a question that must be addressed. Powell ends her chapter with this statement:

> We haven't done a great job as a society of tackling obvious risks related to sex, driving, and money—and those are just the problems we know about. We'll need to do better. Finding the right balance between freedom and safety is hard in dementia and in life. Looking for sources of joy and watching out for obvious risks starts us off on the path to a good life with dementia.[32]

I would add one thorny issue to Powell's list: guns. This is definitely a third rail issue in the US because of persistent controversy over various forms of gun control (for example, requiring background checks, having a mandatory waiting period for gun purchases, and forbidding purchase of military-style weapons). Three recent papers have addressed approaches to gun ownership and use by people living with dementia.

A study published in 2011 used data from the Veterans Administration over a five-year period for nearly 300,000 persons age 60 and older having dementia. Of the 241 persons in the sample who died by suicide, 73 percent used guns. Comorbidities of depression or anxiety increased the suicide risk, in addition to availability of firearms.[33] Not only is suicide a concern for persons having dementia with access to guns, but families and caregivers may also be at risk of injury or death. The authors of a paper on how clinicians should assess risk compared it to assessments of driving. They urged families of persons having dementia who also have firearms to consider a kind of advance directive both for driving and for firearm use. They included an example with the paper. It states that the person recognizes that a time might come when it would be no longer possible to make good decisions about owning and using guns (or about driving), and it designates a trusted person to take necessary steps to ensure safety while also respecting dignity and rights.[34]

A 2014 paper published in Australia compared firearm regulation and use in Australia and the US. Firearm ownership is significantly less common in Australia than in the US, and the regulations are stricter. Although there are variations in how each state and territory in Australia regulates gun ownership, in general all require a minimum delay of 28 days between applying for a permit to purchase a gun and receiving permission. This has reduced suicide rates in people age 55 and older. The authors of this paper offered specific suggestions for clinicians in making capacity assessments of people having dementia. In some persons, dementia symptoms may not affect their ability to understand the responsibilities of firearm ownership and use; other persons, however, may no longer be able to engage in complex decision-making. The paper's authors recommended a combination of capacity assessment and risk assessment, the latter focusing on mental-health issues.[35]

All of these difficult issues need to be addressed by communities that want to be dementia friendly. Who should determine when sexual relations by persons having dementia are inappropriate? How should states regulate who can operate a motor vehicle safely? How should financial institutions and families respond when people having dementia insist on managing their money? Who should assess whether people with dementia should have access to guns? To help people answer these questions, the Joseph Rowntree

Foundation (JRF) sponsored a study of positive risk-taking in dementia-friendly communities. This is the same organization that has promoted the Four Cornerstones Model for creating dementia-friendly communities. Their report on positive risk-taking employed a strengths-based approach that affirms and supports the dignity of people living with dementia. It emphasizes what people can do rather than what they cannot do and states that decisions about risk need to be made on the basis of understanding the presence or absence of a person's strengths. Importantly, this paper emphasizes that in dementia-friendly communities "more people share the perceived burden or responsibilities for care and support and challenge fears about giving more power and choice to people living with dementia."[36]

These questions about risk require careful study by people from various professional backgrounds collaborating with people living with dementia. They also need to be framed within the context of a progressive condition such that an individual might be perfectly safe to drive or use a gun now, but that this could change in a year. With the rapid maturation of the movement toward dementia-friendly communities, all of these issues urgently need our attention.

Fortunately, guidance for thinking about what JRF calls "positive risk-taking," otherwise known as "negotiated risk,"[37] is becoming more widely available. Generally, these resources note the high level of risk aversion among professionals and organizations that work with people having dementia. Obviously they need to be concerned about preventing personal injury, but they also want to avoid organizational liability and unwanted media attention. Unfortunately, risk aversion can quickly lead to a diminishment of dignity for people with dementia when they are no longer permitted to exercise any autonomy or agency.

Decisions by family members and professionals about how to balance the risks and benefits of allowing choices will vary depending on the person and the situation. Everyone needs to understand the benefits a person would obtain from a risky behavior (an example could be as mundane as taking a walk in a neighborhood) compared with the potential harm. A plan needs to be made that everyone agrees upon, because something like a fall will affect not only the individual with dementia but also care partners, plus organizations if the individual resides in a care community. Like JRF, most authors addressing this difficult issue of risk management advocate for a strengths-based approach that affirms what the person with dementia can do instead of what the person cannot do.

Communities committed to being dementia friendly can support people with dementia and their families in making decisions about risk. For example, they should ensure that local emergency services and law-enforcement personnel are trained in appropriate and helpful ways to respond to people with dementia. The whole community should be educated about dementia and the social model of disability. That model would emphasize a collaborative approach to decision-making about risk that includes to the extent possible the person with dementia. This is not easy by any means. But it can be done.

An outstanding example of what can happen when the idea of positive risk-taking is embraced comes from the work of the British organization Dementia Adventure.[38] As stated on the homepage of its website, its goal is to help people living with dementia retain a sense of adventure by getting outdoors and connecting with nature, themselves, and their community. To support this goal, the organization organizes all kinds of holidays for families in various locations in England. Dementia Adventure even sponsors multi-day sailing trips.

Conclusion

Dementia-friendly and inclusive communities happen not because someone completed a checklist but because people living with dementia were asked what would make for a good life and then were invited to participate in planning and carrying out activities to support as good a life as possible. These communities offer hope, not in the form of a miracle cure but in the kind acts of neighbors, the helpful responses of shopkeepers, the support and respite offered to care partners, and the engagement of people of all ages interacting with individuals whose diagnosis still evokes such dread in many people. People living in these communities are unafraid to engage with the difficult third-rail issues mentioned in this chapter. These are communities of people who do not deny the many difficult challenges of dementia but always affirm possibilities for enduring, meaningful relationships throughout the dementia journey, relationships that support the dignity of everyone who lives with dementia. As the next two chapters demonstrate, many communities have discovered that programs focusing on creative engagement and the arts, as well as various ways of honoring spiritual connections, can significantly enhance life quality for people living with dementia.

Endnotes

1   World Health Organization. (2007). *Global age-friendly cities: A guide.* Geneva, Switzerland: World Health Organization. Accessed on 7/23/19 at www.who.int/ageing/publications/Global_age_friendly_cities_Guide_English.pdf

2   Thomas, W. H., & Blanchard, J. M. (2009). Moving beyond place: Aging in community. *Generations, 33*(2), 12–17.

3   Innovations in Dementia. (2011). *Dementia capable communities: The views of people with dementia and their supporters.* Exeter, UK: Innovations in Dementia. Accessed on 7/23/19 at www.housinglin.org.uk/_assets/Resources/Housing/OtherOrganisation/DementiaCapableCommunities_fullreportFeb2011.pdf

4   Innovations in Dementia, p. 8.

5   Innovations in Dementia, p. 8.

6   Innovations in Dementia, p. 19.

7   Green, G. (2013). *Building dementia-friendly communities: A priority for everyone.* London, UK: Alzheimer's Society. Accessed on 7/23/19 at www.actonalz.org/sites/default/files/documents/Dementia_friendly_communities_full_report.pdf

8   The 2009 National Dementia Strategy is notable for many reasons, beginning with what is expressed on its cover page. That page contains photographs of a number of smiling people with the subheading "Putting People First": Department of Health. (2009). *Living well with dementia: A national dementia strategy.* London, UK: Department of Health. Accessed on 6/25/19 at https://assets.publishing.service.gov.uk/government/uploads/system/uploads/attachment_data/file/168221/dh_094052.pdf

    Compare that with the dull, bureaucratic document issued by the US Department of Health and Human Services in 2012. Note also the difference between producing a plan focusing on dementia in general and one that names only Alzheimer's: US Department of Health and Human Services. (2012). *National plan to address Alzheimer's disease.* Washington, DC: US Department of Health and Human Services. Accessed on 6/25/19 at https://aspe.hhs.gov/system/files/pdf/102526/NatlPlan2012%20with%20Note.pdf

9   Henwood, C., & Downs, M. (2014). Dementia-friendly communities. In M. Downs & B. Bowers (Eds.), *Excellence in dementia care: Research into practice* (2nd ed., pp. 20–35). Maidenhead, UK: Open University Press.

10 Heward, M., Innes, A., Cutler, C., & Hambidge, S. (2016). Dementia-friendly communities: Challenges and strategies for achieving stakeholder involvement. *Health and Social Care in the Community, 25,* 858–867.

11 www.dfamerica.org/what-is-dfa

12 For more information about the Dementia Friends program, see: www.dfamerica. org/dementia-friends-usa

13 Hebert, C. A., & Scales, K. (2017). Dementia friendly initiatives: A state of the science review. *Dementia, 18*(5), 1858–1895. (p. 1887)

14 Alzheimer Europe. (2015). *Dementia in Europe yearbook 2015: Is Europe becoming more dementia friendly?* Luxembourg: Alzheimer Europe. Available via www. alzheimer-europe.org/Publications/Dementia-in-Europe-Yearbooks

15 In 2018, FVMP became an independent, nonprofit organization. When it began in 2012, it was affiliated with Lutheran Social Services of Wisconsin and Upper Michigan as its fiscal agent. The FVMP website has information about its mission and values as well as descriptions of its programs and calendars of cafés and other social gatherings: www.foxvalleymemoryproject.org

16 McFadden, S. H., & McFadden, J. T. (2011). *Aging together: Dementia, friendship, and flourishing communities.* Baltimore, MD: Johns Hopkins University Press.

17 Sedensky, M. (2018, December 5). "It's like 'Mean Girls' but everyone is 80": How nursing homes deal with bullies. *USA Today.* Accessed on 7/10/19 at www. usatoday.com/story/news/nation/2018/05/12/nursing-homes-senior-centers-bullying/604758002

    Span, P. (2011, May 31). Mean girls in assisted living. *New York Times New Old Age blog.* Accessed on 7/10/19 at https://newoldage.blogs.nytimes.com/2011/05/31/mean-girls-in-the-nursing-home

    Weiner, J. (2015, January 18). Mean girls in the retirement home. *New York Times,* p. SR4. Accessed on 7/10/19 at www.nytimes.com/2015/01/18/opinion/sunday/mean-girls-in-the-retirement-home.html

18 Bonifas, R. P. (2016). *Bullying among older adults: How to recognize and address an unseen epidemic.* Baltimore, MD: Health Professions Press.

19 Cahill, S. (2018). *Dementia and human rights.* Chicago, IL: Policy Press. (p. 96)

20 As noted at the beginning of Chapter 5, people with younger-onset dementia in the US can qualify for Social Security Disability Insurance, although many people have no idea this is possible.

21 Roach, P., & Drummond, N. (2014). "It's nice to have something to do": Early-onset dementia and maintaining purposeful activity. *Journal of Psychiatric and Mental Health Nursing, 21,* 889–895.

22 Black, S. E., Gauthier, S., Dalziel, W., Keren, R., Correia, J., Hew, H., & Binder, C. (2010). Canadian Alzheimer's disease caregiver survey: Baby-boomer caregivers and burden of care. *International Journal of Geriatric Psychiatry, 25,* 807–813.

23 In the US, the third rail is the rail with electric current that powers subway trains. Touch it, and you die, or at least suffer terrible injuries. It generally refers to issues people—especially politicians—do not want to address.

24 Shaw, G. (December, 2011/January, 2012). Dementia in the workplace. *Neurology Now, 8*(6), 30–33.

25 The Wisconsin Department of Health Services produced an employer toolkit aimed at helping organizations support dementia care-partners: www.dhs.wisconsin.gov/dementia/employers.htm

26 Polivka, L., & Luo, B. (2019). Neoliberal long-term care: From community to corporate control. *The Gerontologist, 59,* 222–229. (p. 227)

27 Post, S. (2000). *The moral challenge of Alzheimer disease: Ethical issues from diagnosis to dying* (2nd ed.). Baltimore, MD: Johns Hopkins University Press.

28 Henig, R. M. (2015, May 17). The last day. *New York Times Magazine*, p. 36. Accessed on 9/28/19 at www.nytimes.com/2015/05/17/magazine/the-last-day-of-her-life.html

29 Kellehear, A. (2009). Dementia and dying: The need for a systematic policy approach. *Critical Social Policy, 29*, 146–157. (p. 150)

30 Sampson, E. L., & Robinson, L. (Eds.). (2009). End of life care in dementia [Special issue]. *Dementia, 8*(3).

31 Powell, T. (2019). *Dementia reimagined: Building a life of joy and dignity from beginning to end.* New York: NY: Avery.

32 Powell, p. 247.

33 Seyfried, L. S., Kales, H. C., Ignacio, R. V., Conwell, Y., & Valenstein, M. (2011). *Alzheimer's & Dementia, 7*, 567–573.

34 Betz, M. E., McCourt, A. D., Vernick, J. S., Ranney, M. L., Maust, D. T., & Wintemute, G. J. (2018). Firearms and dementia: Clinical considerations. *Annals of Internal Medicine, 169*, 47–49.

35 Wand, A. P. F., Pelsah, C., Strukovski, J-A., & Brodaty, H. (2014). Firearms, mental illness, dementia, and the clinician. *Medical Journal of Australia, 201*, 674–678.

36 Morgan, S., & Williamson, T. (2014). *How can "positive risk-taking" help build dementia-friendly communities?* York, UK: Joseph Rowntree Foundation. (p. 10). Accessed on 4/14/20 at www.jrf.org.uk/report/how-can-positive-risk-taking-help-build-dementia-friendly-communities

37 Dr. Allen Power's book on well-being in persons having dementia identifies seven domains of well-being: identity, connectedness, security, autonomy, meaning, growth, and joy. In the chapter on autonomy, he discusses the concept of negotiated risk: Power, G. A. (2014). *Dementia beyond disease: Enhancing well-being.* Baltimore, MD: Health Professions Press.

38 https://dementiaadventure.co.uk

Part 4

CREATIVITY AND THE HUMAN SPIRIT

Chapter 9

Arts and Artists in Dementia-Friendly and Inclusive Communities

People who have edited themselves into silence for fear of saying the wrong thing, or shut themselves down to avoid contact they cannot understand, can use the arts to reconnect with themselves and the people who care for them. And perhaps most important, the arts offer a chance for people with dementia to connect with the people who have forgotten them—their communities at large.

—Anne Basting[1]

As my husband, John, and I walked toward the entrance to a nursing home in eastern Kentucky, we heard a man calling out, "Come and get your wings!" Dressed in a red sports coat, Bermuda shorts, a floral shirt, two neckties, and a funny hat, this jovial man was standing outside the front doors, handing out wings that were cut from white paper plates and attached to pieces of yarn so they could be worn around the neck. Later, we learned that this man had some acting experience but, in his day job, served as the county executive and the county judge.

John and I had road-tripped from Wisconsin, and our son and daughter-in-law had arrived the day before from Minnesota, all of us intent on experiencing a play in a rural nursing-home care community where nearly all residents were supported through the Medicaid program. *Wendy's Neverland*, a retelling of the Peter Pan story from the perspective of Wendy as an older woman in hospice care at a nursing home, was in its second day of performances. Standing outside the building (a typical 1960s single-story nursing home with several wings of its own) was a group of over 60 people of all ages, waiting to be invited in to witness a remarkable transformation.

How do you turn a traditional nursing home into a lively, engaging place where residents and staff delight in a performance for community members (and a few visitors from far away) that overflows with joy and meaning? The TimeSlips nonprofit organization has figured out how to do work that is almost magical in its effects on everyone involved. With grants to Kentucky from the Civil Money Penalties program (fines collected for Medicare and Medicaid fraud and abuse), TimeSlips staff collaborated with Signature HealthCARE, local and national artists, and residents and staff of 12 Kentucky nursing homes to create a play featuring pirates, lost boys and girls, a crocodile, and an old woman whose wondrous stories of adventures with these characters are not believed because, well, she is old and she has dementia. The play was performed at three of the nursing homes, each of which had worked closely with three others in their region.

Wendy's story emerged from several years of structured discussions with residents about what they would like to tell Peter— the boy who said he would never grow up—about what they had lost and what they had gained in their own experiences of growing up and older. In other words, the whole project—from the early workshops to create the story to the final production—was dementia inclusive. Working with local bluegrass musicians, visual artists, a choreographer from Chicago, and a Kentucky-based actor/director, residents and staff created an immersive theater experience that had the audience laughing, weeping, dancing, and singing along with people living with dementia and other disabilities severe enough to require skilled nursing care.

After putting on our wings, we entered the nursing home and were invited to express our fears about aging by writing them on canning jar lids the residents had decorated. Later, in the rehab therapy room, the audience gathered to watch Captain Hook feed our fears to the Croc; they became part of his spiky tail. We also wrote happy images of our own aging on pieces of paper shaped like clouds, clouds that were then attached to string to float gently above us.

As we walked through the nursing home, following the characters in the play and interacting with residents, staff, and a few community members, including children—all in colorful costumes and face paint—we saw that every hallway was decorated with images expressing parts of Wendy's Neverland. In a large activity room, we listened to recordings of residents' voices as they related what they would like to tell Peter about what they had gained and lost. Another scene took place in the dining room where we received "flying" lessons by learning movements with our arms. In one of my favorite moments, I interacted with a woman using a wheelchair as we joyfully sang "I'll Fly Away" with the musicians, residents, staff, and the rest of the audience.

As the play drew to an end, we gathered again in the dining area for a remarkable wheelchair ballet featuring 12 residents moving to music and instructions from the Croc, an actor wearing a huge crocodile head and a long tail from which its sharp spikes—our fears—had fallen. He stood in the middle of the circle calling out the moves to the staff and family members pushing the wheelchairs. Then the Croc and Wendy (a resident using a wheelchair) spoke movingly about friendship and her imminent death. Residents and staff honored Wendy by saying how much her stories had meant to them; and as the play concluded, Wendy rose from her wheelchair and walked quietly out of the room. We all knew she was walking toward death, but also that her stories would be treasured for ever. Wendy was believed. Something powerful and important had happened in Wendy's Neverland: we had been invited to believe the residents who told us their names and shared their stories about what growing up and older had taught them.[2]

Celebrating Creativity

I should disclose here that I chaired the board of directors of TimeSlips for six years and have been involved in various ways with TimeSlips since 2003, including as a certified facilitator of the TimeSlips creative-storytelling method.

TimeSlips has grown to be an internationally acclaimed organization, reaching people through its trainings in the storytelling method for families, community members, and residential-care staff, and through teaching high-school and college students to connect with elders through storytelling and other art forms. A third component of TimeSlips focuses on helping long-term care residences like the ones in Kentucky become Creative Communities of Care (the CCC model). Through all of these programs for "connecting through creativity," TimeSlips aims to positively reframe aging and dementia care and to bring meaning and purpose to elders through creative engagement.[3]

Wendy's Neverland is an example of how TimeSlips teaches creative engagement with elders, encourages community members to connect meaningfully with long-term care residents, and celebrates the strengths of people having dementia and other conditions commonly associated with aging. This emphasis on celebrations is one of the most important elements of TimeSlips' work. This means that whether nursing assistants trained in skilled care are creating stories with residents using the TimeSlips method, or organizations have embraced the CCC model and have engaged with artists to create a theatrical production such as *Wendy's Neverland*, the public is always invited to witness and celebrate the results.

One important element of the CCC model is its training for introducing creative engagement into the ordinary care practices and activities of long-term care as well as the tasks of care partners in private homes. For example, picture a nursing aide helping a resident dress in the morning. She has many residents to attend to in a limited amount of time, so the default approach is to be friendly but efficient so she can move on to the next resident. However, an ordinary interaction like this could be a platform for a creative exchange. In the time it takes to help someone put on a shirt and a sweater, she could say something like "What beautiful sound would you like to hear today?" To answer this question requires no memory, and there are no wrong answers. It is an example of what the TimeSlips organization calls a "beautiful question." It could just as easily be a question asked by a husband helping his wife get dressed in the morning.

Residential care communities of all types usually have at least one staff person whose job description calls for organizing activities.

Sometimes these activities are described as offering "life enrichment." However, too often they are dull, repetitious, and only minimally able to engage curiosity and evoke communication from people with dementia. By training staff in various types of creative-engagement activities—such as creating poems, songs, stories, and art works—these communities emphasize the joys of co-creation. The example of *Wendy's Neverland* shows that these activities do not have to be one-time-only events, but rather they can be integrated into a long-term, collaborative project that can go in many directions depending on the inspiration of residents and staff.

A few years ago, before the CCC model was fully developed, Fox Valley Memory Project (FVMP) in Wisconsin received a grant to train nursing assistants from 10 care communities in the TimeSlips storytelling method. After each care community had collected stories over the course of several months, they selected their favorite stories, and from them, they constructed buildings for a "TimeSlips Town" using enormous pieces of cardboard. With the help of some high-school students, we set up the town in a large room in a local senior center and invited the community to come for an afternoon to interact with residents, see their creative productions, and sit in our "diner" to enjoy free pieces of warm apple pie donated by a local bakery. In addition to the diner, we had a pet shop, shoe store, ice cream parlor, superheroes comic-book shop, library, lemonade stand, and "grandma's front porch." All were based on stories residents of the care communities had created. Everyone who attended got a booklet containing these stories and the photographs that had inspired them.

Events like these remove socially reinforced barriers between those having dementia and people of all ages sharing the same community. Whether such events involve people in Kentucky following an actor wearing a giant crocodile costume as he spins a story with residents at a rural Medicaid nursing home, or people in Wisconsin gathering on a Saturday afternoon for imaginative fun and apple pie, they demonstrate that people with dementia can contribute to the wider community through their creativity—*they do not need to remember, because they can still imagine.* In addition, they are given an important social role—actor, singer, artist, dancer, storyteller—that enriches the lives of family members, friends, and people who just wander in to find out what all the excitement is about.

During the TimeSlips Town program, I witnessed the happy engagement of people with dementia and care partners I know through FVMP memory cafés. Here was an afternoon of fun and neighborly connections created by people living with dementia in long-term care, places to which café participants eventually may need to relocate. The usual mantra of "nursing homes are terrible places, and I'd never want to live in one" was absent because that day demonstrated possibilities for infusing creativity into the lives of those who live and work in long-term care.

There are many other ways for arts celebrations to connect long-term care residents having more advanced dementia with those living with dementia in their homes and with community members. For example, FVMP organized a poetry party using skills taught by Gary Glazner of the Alzheimer's Poetry Project.[4] Long-term care residents and community members with dementia gathered with care staff, home-based care partners, and people from the wider community to participate in call-and-response recitation of well-known poems and to hear new poems created by residents.

FVMP sponsors these arts celebrations annually. One year, middle-school students in an art class received basic instruction about dementia and then teamed with memory-care residents and people living at home with dementia for an afternoon of story sharing and the co-creation of drawings. Another time, an art show displayed the works of residents from several care communities at an event that also featured a chorus of people with dementia and care partners. That art show included a large grouping of mosaics created by people with dementia living at home with care partners who attended a program at a local art museum. And as a last example, FVMP received a small grant for a man who describes himself as a "rhythm facilitator" to teach staff from several care communities how to create drum rhythms with residents. We then gathered residents who had practiced their rhythms on simple instruments made by memory café participants from wood and packing tape. Picture a large room with about 150 people—all ages, all levels of cognitive ability—drumming along to the song "We Will Rock You." All of these celebrations connected children and adults, and people with and without dementia, for the pure pleasure of experiencing how the arts can unite people regardless of cognitive status.

Programs like these are proliferating around the world, springing from the energy and imagination of artists, theatrical companies, residential care communities, foundations, researchers, universities, and even medical organizations. For example, the University of Washington's Memory and Brain Wellness Center collaborated with the University of British Columbia's Centre for Research on Personhood in Dementia to organize the 2019 Dementia Without Borders festival.[5] It happened at the Peace Arch Provincial Park, an international park consisting of Peace Arch Historical State Park in Washington State and Peace Arch Provincial Park in British Columbia. Hundreds of people from the United States and Canada could cross the border without passports and enjoy a day of music, poetry, paintings, film, dance, and other art forms. Boundaries were erased, not only between the two countries but also between people often separated by fear and stigma: people having dementia living in residential care, people with dementia living in their homes, and community members of all ages. Rejecting the common tragedy narrative rooted in medical descriptions of diseased brains and impaired cognition, this celebration of creativity lifted up images of dignity and hope.

Such affirmation of the social citizenship of people living with dementia represented a key organizing principle for the Dementia Without Borders celebration. As Chapter 3 noted, the idea of social citizenship is a relatively new construct among researchers and practitioners. Unlike the traditional approach to citizenship, which focuses on individual rights and responsibilities, the social citizenship model emphasizes practices and relationships that secure fundamental rights. These include the right of an individual to grow in relation with others who affirm the person as whole (not just a person having a disease), to be free of discrimination, and to exercise agency in their lives.[6]

Agency means that people living with all types of dementia, and at all stages, are welcomed to express who they are and what they desire. If agency cannot be communicated with words, it can be communicated through gestures, sounds, facial expressions, and creative engagement.[7] Dementia Without Borders, TimeSlips Town,

Wendy's Neverland, and other arts-based projects like these enable people to remain included in their communities—communities committed to the idea that dementia does not eliminate the human need for meaning and purpose. Relationships in these inclusive communities that celebrate the artistic expressions of people with dementia encourage all kinds of expressions of agency. For example, those who need assistance in communicating who they are and what they desire can receive support when someone teaches them a dance motion, hands them a paintbrush and paper, or encourages them to contribute to the creation of a story.

Why Do This?

A few years ago, Canadian researcher Sherry Dupuis and three colleagues participated in an arts-based workshop along with people having dementia, family members, and visual and performance artists. Their day of art making focused on exploring alternatives to the tragedy discourse of decline and deterioration. The researchers asked how that discourse affected people living with dementia, how those persons wanted others' views of them to change, and what they thought people should know about what it is like to experience dementia either as a diagnosed person or care partner.

After a morning spent discussing these questions, the participants divided into small groups, with each group including a visual or performance artist, a researcher, and people with dementia and family members. Their assignment was to work collaboratively on an artistic presentation of the lived experience of dementia. They painted, wrote poetry, and created brief performances that challenged the dominant discourse. Later, the researchers conducted telephone interviews with everyone who participated in the workshop, including the researchers themselves, to find out how the workshop had affected them.

The project had emerged from a commitment to critically address the social-justice issues raised by the tragedy narrative about dementia. The researchers wanted to demonstrate how the arts can help us engage with issues of justice for people living with dementia "in accessible and emotional ways, opening up new ways of seeing, and broadening understanding."[8] Inspired by the work of Clive

Baldwin of the Bradford Dementia Group in the United Kingdom and what he refers to as the "narrative citizenship" of people living with dementia, the researchers tested whether his ideas could be affirmed through arts participation.[9]

Narrative citizenship means that people have the *right* to tell their own stories—acts Baldwin describes as expressions of narrative agency. By telling their own stories through various art forms, people can experience growth as they discover that their stories matter to others. Although they may initially think that they have nothing meaningful to contribute, by working with skillful, patient, and understanding arts mentors they often discover they have quite a lot that can be shared and valued by other people. This work can provide a self-portrait of their uniqueness, give a sense of purpose, and demonstrate agency.

Baldwin suggests three approaches to understanding the narrative agency of people with dementia. First, he states that whether or not they can communicate verbally, they can be invited to express themselves through arts participation. Second, communication implies some kind of relationship; we employ narrative agency when we co-construct our stories with others—just as Wendy and the Croc did. Finally, the narrative agency of one person can become part of another's story. Thus, we can imagine the Croc someday describing how he and Wendy became friends and how she became a character in his story.

When Dupuis and her fellow researchers held the workshop with people having dementia, family members, and artists, they embraced all three of these expressions of narrative agency. Through visual and performance arts, the participants related how they felt about the dominant view of dementia, and they formed relationships with researchers and artists by sharing these feelings. Interviews with the artists and researchers revealed how these stories affected them. One artist described the experience like this:

> The participants left with something, [and] I left with something, so there was an exchange, as opposed to I'm here and I'm going to give you stuff and walk away totally drained! I didn't walk away with the feeling "I gave my time for something great!" I walked away with personal change.[10]

Reflecting a similar feeling, a researcher said, "I'm suddenly a different person forever for having experienced this… [I] will never forget."[11]

The transformational process also affected people having dementia. For example, one participant commented, "[It] reinforced me in my efforts to teach everyone that there is life after diagnosis. I need to keep on teaching everyone I meet. The workshop has given me a real boost in knowing that we can make a difference."[12] Similarly, a family member described being affected by hearing stories from other family members about advocacy within their communities to change the typical dementia narrative.

The way that they made art with others—art that expressed feelings about having dementia and how others view people living with it—ended up being transformative for everyone who participated. Researchers got in touch with their own vulnerabilities, an unusual outcome because of the psychological distance ordinarily enforced between people doing research and the people they are studying. Family members recognized new possibilities for self-expression in their loved ones. Artists witnessed the power of their arts to shift narratives and create relationships. People with dementia discovered that they could overcome their shame about their diagnosis by telling their stories through different art forms. The workshop and the insights gathered from the subsequent interviews amply demonstrated "the relational and emancipatory potential of the arts."[13]

The Arts and Attitude Change

Arts programs of many different kinds are spreading throughout the world as more people embrace the idea that the fundamental rights of citizenship and narrative agency should not be denied just because a person has some kind of dementia diagnosis. Indeed, as the work of Dupuis and her colleagues demonstrated, arts participation and opportunities for creative engagement can be transformational for people having dementia, their care partners and friends, artists, and even researchers. Sharing these creative expressions in community celebrations such as *Wendy's Neverland*, TimeSlips Town, and Dementia Without Borders offers opportunities for transformations to occur in public attitudes about dementia.

Because the arts speak to people in emotional and symbolic languages, art may be more effective in changing attitudes than lectures accompanied by wordy PowerPoint slides. This idea has been amply supported by the German sociologist Verena Rothe, who has described numerous exhibitions of paintings, films, plays, and other artistic expression happening in Germany in recent years, all featuring works by people with dementia. She says:

> Art and cultural events reach groups of people who would not necessarily come to a lecture or an activist meeting. At the same time, the creative domains, bringing together a wide range of perspectives, can hopefully give rise to new ideas and unfamiliar experimental approaches different from those that focus on professional care structures.[14]

But of course, it is the professional care structures that have so much influence on the lives of everyone affected by dementia: diagnosed persons, care partners, paid caregivers, medical professionals, and community members. These care structures rely on scientific affirmation of the value and worth of actions usually labeled as "interventions"—actions or policies designed to improve a situation. Therefore, we must ask: Is there any valid, reliable evidence regarding how arts practices affect people with dementia, care partners, paid caregivers, medical professionals, artists, and their communities?

Where's the Evidence?

Imagine going to your doctor with a really sore throat. The examination and swab test indicate that you have strep throat, and based on her knowledge of the scientific literature and experience treating others with this condition, the doctor may prescribe an antibiotic. She may be concerned that leaving the infection untreated could lead to rheumatic fever or other serious complications. She knows there is considerable evidence accumulated over many years about the effectiveness of certain antibiotics for strep throat, as well as research showing the dangers of antibiotic over-prescription.

Now imagine that you were diagnosed with Alzheimer's dementia two years ago. You have managed pretty well, but over the last year your spouse has noticed that you have become more withdrawn and forgetful. You seldom leave your house. Today you go to your primary care doctor for your annual check-up. Your spouse comes with you and reports your lack of energy and unwillingness to do anything but watch television. How will your doctor respond? Will he prescribe an antidepressant? Maybe. Will he suggest some cognitive tests? Hopefully. But, if you live in the UK, your doctor might also urge you to participate in a local singing group for people with dementia and care partners once a week in the community center. Your own doctor, if you are fortunate, might recommend an arts program regularly offered at a nearby museum. In other words, your doctor might prescribe some kind of engagement with the arts. He would know that these programs "provide access to connection with friends, family, and extended community and access to ways of giving meaning to experiences, feelings, and observations."[15]

Arts prescribing (sometimes called Arts on Prescription, or AoP), a specific form of the more broadly defined act of social prescribing (which can include social activities ranging from card playing to volunteering), has been happening in the UK since the 1990s[16] and has spread to Norway, Denmark, and Sweden.[17] These arts programs differ from those led by certified arts therapists working in hospitals, nursing homes, or other settings where they can receive reimbursement for their work as an evidence-based medical treatment. Arts programs, ranging in size and complexity from a project such as *Wendy's Neverland* to a regular volunteer bringing his ukulele to sing with nursing-home residents, do not claim to be medical treatments; rather, they focus on eliciting joy, encouraging social connectedness, and showing that meaning can be infused into everyday life for people living with dementia.

According to the National Coalition of Creative Art Therapies Associations, poetry, dance, visual art, psychodrama, music, and drama therapies have empirically demonstrated outcomes such as "improving communication and expression, and increasing physical, emotional, cognitive and/or social functioning."[18] Therapists working with these art forms need to be able to demonstrate effectiveness in terms of achievement of specific goals. Their professional organizations and certified training programs know this work is supported by many years of research showing significant, measurable improvements particularly for persons having mental-health issues.

Poets, dancers, visual artists, musicians, actors, and others who work with people with dementia, family members, and volunteers in venues such as memory cafés, art galleries, museums, and community centers, as well as with staff in residential care communities, also believe that their work has positive outcomes. Although they may not use this language, in effect they are helping to improve communication and interpersonal relationships by supporting narrative agency through creative expression. They observe participants' increased social interaction in their programs as they become more comfortable with the group and its activities. They may be aware that evidence is mounting that demonstrates improvements in mood and engagement with others. They do not claim that their work is a substitute for medical interventions, rather that it can be allied with them. In some countries, it can be reimbursed.

As these arts practices with people having dementia have been embraced worldwide, there have been increasing calls for researchers to use the "gold standard" of medical intervention studies: studies that randomly assign people to groups, administer a treatment to one group and a placebo-type treatment to another group, and then compare them using measuring instruments with proven validity and reliability.[19] However, for many reasons, this is challenging for arts and health researchers who may be able to randomly assign groups but struggle to obtain groups of study participants large enough to meet statistical requirements.[20] Often the solution is to use a "pre–post" design, meaning that they take measurements before beginning the arts program and then again when it ends, sometimes even returning several months later for another round of data collection.

In addition to the difficulty of designing a study with random assignment to groups, consider the difference between being in a medical study, in which you may get a placebo (like a sugar pill) or a drug without knowing which group you are in, and being in a study of some kind of creative engagement, in which you know you are painting with an artist who is helping you by providing supplies and encouragement. Psychologists have repeatedly demonstrated that if research participants know they are in a group expected to perform in a certain way, participants may meet those expectations not because the treatment is so effective but because they are happy to be in the group and want to please the researcher. Psychologists also know that researchers themselves can influence outcomes if they know that one group is expected to do better than another group. This is why the gold standard also calls for researchers to be "blind" to the group assignments and for participants to be "blind" to their assigned group. This approach is simply not possible for most people trying to do scientifically sound evaluations of creative-engagement programs.

The answer to the question "where's the evidence?" of the effectiveness of arts programs for people with dementia also hinges on the method of data collection, as well as design issues. A commonly used method—called qualitative research—employs observations and/or interviews that are carefully analyzed using structured approaches that have been shown to produce valid, reliable evidence. This was the approach taken by Dupuis and her colleagues when they developed the workshop for people with dementia, care partners, artists, and researchers. However, qualitative research is not acceptable to some critics who note that this research is riddled with confounding problems like an absence of the random assignment and blinded observers and participants found in clinical trials of medical interventions. Despite many solid arguments for the scientific soundness of qualitative methods, there remains suspicion among some that the only research that counts is research with data that can be submitted to various statistical tests.

Even in light of these challenges, we should not give up on attempting to do research on arts practices with people having dementia. In addition, as we will observe in several examples below, it is possible to collect numerical data using standardized tests.[21] Often this kind of data is required for programs to receive grant funding to support this work.

Many possible outcomes of creative engagement with various art forms have been investigated. A common goal of creative engagement is to produce improvement in people's perceived quality of life. There are several well-documented ways of measuring this, one of the most popular being the QoL-AD scale.[22] A comparison of research on pharmacologic, psychosocial, and cultural arts "interventions" found that, except for the administration of donepezil (Aricept), there was little evidence from research on pharmacologic approaches of significant, positive effects on quality of life. Psychosocial interventions such as behavior modification (rewarding positive behaviors and withholding rewards for less desirable behaviors) and activities tailored to a person's interests and capacities also produced an increased sense of quality of life. Other pharmacologic and psychosocial interventions did reduce anxiety, wandering, and behaviors generally described as problematic by care partners and care staff, but they did not have an effect on the person's overall quality of life. In comparison, there were strong indications that the cultural arts programs produced pleasure, an improved quality of life, and better communication.

The authors of this review argued that in order to understand how participation in arts programs can help people with dementia live as well as possible, new study designs and measures are required.[23] They urged researchers to stop trying to compare, for example, outcomes of dancing to outcomes of painting, but rather to understand in general *how* cultural arts programs work to improve life quality and well-being. They also urged that attention be paid not only to the individual with dementia but also to the ways that arts practices affect family members, staff, and people in the community. Another way of thinking about this is to say that the loneliness, helplessness, and boredom too often experienced by people having dementia—regardless of the type or progression of the condition—need to be addressed by considering the effects of arts participation on the person's social context and interactions with other people. Arts programs are social; they can elicit and nurture relationality.

As noted in another detailed review of the literature on arts programs and persons having dementia, much of the research focuses on measuring reductions in what some label as "behavioral and psychological symptoms of dementia" (BPSDs) measured by objective scales completed by trained observers. Again, the focus is on the individual, and the measures address what disturbs or annoys other people, not what supports a more enjoyable and meaningful life for the person with dementia. These studies usually take place in residential care communities where those with advanced dementia are more likely to live. It is certainly true that people living in these communities do engage in these behaviors, usually because that may be their only way of communicating distress, pain, or some other troubling issue. Fewer studies attempt to obtain indications of changes in participants' overall subjective feelings of well-being, their enjoyment of the activity, and the ways arts participation supports social interaction. Also, much of this research does not include people living with earlier stages of the dementia process.[24]

Sometimes research on arts involvement focuses not on the person making the art but on the creative product. Some might say that the individual appeared to have fun during the art-making session but produced a mess of a painting. This is an old debate in creativity research, one that Paul Camic and his colleagues argued needs to be retired and replaced by emphasizing "process and experience" instead of product. Also, when the individual works with another person to create something ("co-creativity"), Camic and colleagues state that "components such as mutual endeavor, relational interactions, and notions of shared creativity"[25] are added and may be more important than the end product of the creative-engagement process. These can be measured and are particularly significant because they place

> less emphasis and demand on production and end point measurement, whilst giving more attention to encouraging enjoyment, collaboration, exploratory trial and error and discovering what is possible, rather than establishing what is not.[26]

Since the turn of this century, more researchers have been employing what are called "mixed-methods" research designs to gain insight into participants' feelings about being part of these types of creative engagement experiences. This means that they use quantitative measures proven to be valid and reliable, along with qualitative approaches such as interviews that are carefully analyzed for themes and sub-themes. An excellent example comes from an investigation conducted in England and Wales. Over 100 participants were recruited from residential care communities, a county hospital, and community venues (a library, arts center, and an art and music venue). Quantitative and qualitative measurements were taken at the beginning of the study, during the 12-week duration of a weekly, two-hour visual-arts program conducted with small groups, and three and six months after the study ended. In other words, this was a longitudinal study, a rather rare approach in this field. Also, data on the outcomes of interest—observed well-being, quality of life, communication, and participants' perceptions of the sessions—were collected for the arts programs and compared with the control condition of unstructured social activities with no arts components. Overall, the researchers found that participants gave high ratings to their enjoyment of the arts programs. Their scores on measures of well-being, quality of life, and communication also improved (although communication declined in the hospitalized group). Importantly, participants in the arts programs said that the program was "interesting, friendly, and enjoyable" and gave them a "high sense of achievement."[27]

The question many people want to have answered by this research is whether participation in creative-engagement programs will have any effect on the cognitive symptoms of dementia. In other words, might we discover that three months of weekly group singing improves memory, reduces confusion, and increases problem-solving ability, for example? Unfortunately, compared with research on the various forms of art therapy, most of the research I have just discussed does not demonstrate this kind of change. In contrast, arts therapy research has shown positive outcomes for treating conditions such as psychotic episodes, PTSD, depression, anxiety, and other mental-health problems.

Dementia is different. By its very definition it is a progressive condition, so that over the course of the three months of group singing or art making or dancing, there could be declines in scores on cognitive tests because of changes taking place in the brain. Does this mean that the creative engagement was pointless? One can answer yes if one believes that the only thing that matters in dementia is cognitive ability. However, as previous chapters in this book have argued, new ways of thinking about dementia emphasize viewing individuals with the condition as whole persons. Consider how a person with dementia can feel happy long after a particular activity is over. Without relying on words, memory, or reasoning, these new approaches to the arts and dementia emphasize a person's emotional life, as well as the dynamic interactions between people having dementia and their social worlds.

Accumulating research evidence about arts practices shows

positive effects on emotion and social interaction, along with attitudinal changes among care partners, long-term-care staff, medical students, and the general public. The creative-engagement program with the most peer-reviewed empirical support is TimeSlips. Although a person's concept of time does indeed "slip" in the course of dementia, this does not mean that the slipping away of cognitive abilities robs people of opportunities for joyful, meaningful self-expression and meaningful connection with other people.[28]

Research on participation in drama, poetry writing, visual arts, dance, music programs, and combinations of these (as in *Wendy's Neverland*) has been published recently in peer-reviewed journals. The mounting evidence of positive outcomes shown in this research raises the question of when creative-engagement work will be remunerated by health-insurance companies, Medicare, or Medicaid, given the value it brings to so many people.

Artists should not always be expected to volunteer their time and talent. This presents a challenge for the large private corporations that own so many residential care communities, for nonprofits working to improve quality of life, for policy makers who write laws and regulations and oversee budgets, and for families that want the very best for the people they love regardless of where they live, what type(s) of dementia they have, and where they are in the journey. Through the power of the arts, people of all ages, artistic abilities, and cognitive status can come together to tell their stories, laugh and cry together, and experience the joy of celebrating the human spirit of people living with dementia regardless of how advanced the dementia might be. As the next chapter demonstrates, interacting with artists and being encouraged to be creative can be spiritual as well as artistic endeavors.

Endnotes

1   Basting, A. D. (2006). Arts in dementia care: "This is not the end…it's the end of this chapter." *Generations, 30*(1), 16–20. Reproduced with kind permission from the American Society on Aging.

2   For more details about Wendy's Neverland, see: Kramer, E. (2019, July 5). How Kentucky seniors found "Neverland." *American Theatre*. Accessed on 7/20/19 at www.americantheatre.org/2019/07/05/how-kentucky-seniors-found-neverland

See also Anne Basting's recent book: Basting, A. (2020). *Creative care: A revolutionary approach to dementia and elder care.* New York, NY: HarperOne.

Another TimeSlips project involved a continuum-of-care community in Wisconsin that developed a creative collaboration of residents living in all parts of the community, plus participants in its adult day program, along with staff from all parts of the organization from maintenance workers to nurses and administrators. Together with theater students from the University of Wisconsin–Milwaukee and other local artists, they created a play based on the *Odyssey* only told with the focus on Penelope waiting for the return of Odysseus. Details about that project can be found here: Basting, A., Towey, M., & Rose, E. (Eds.). (2016). *The Penelope Project: An arts-based odyssey to change elder care.* Iowa City, IA: University of Iowa Press.

3 www.timeslips.org

4 For videos, sample poems, and more information about the Alzheimer's Poetry Project, see its website:

www.alzpoetry.com

See also: Glazner, G. (2014). *Dementia arts: Celebrating creativity in eldercare.* Baltimore, MD: Health Professions Press.

5 For a detailed description of the Dementia Without Borders day, see: http://depts. washington.edu/mbwc/news/article/dementia-without-borders

6 O'Connor, D., & Netlund, A-C. (2016). Editorial introduction: Special issue on citizenship and dementia. *Dementia, 15*, 285–288.

7 I once participated in a conference in Vancouver, BC, that featured a large, welcoming banner that said, "Art speaks when words fade."

8 Dupuis., S. L., Kontos, P., Mitchell, G., Jonas-Simpson, C., & Gray, J. (2016). Reclaiming citizenship through the arts. *Dementia, 15*, 358–380. (p. 363)

9 Baldwin, C. (2008). Narrative(,) citizenship and dementia: The personal and the political. *Journal of Aging Studies, 22*, 222–228.

10 Dupuis et al., p. 366.

11 Dupuis et al., p. 369.

12 Dupuis et al., p. 369.

13 Dupuis et al., p. 372.

14 Rothe, V. (2017). People in the community living with dementia—the programme. In V. Rothe, G. Kreutzner, & R. Gronemeyer (Eds.), *Staying in life: Paving the way to dementia-friendly communities* (pp. 43–239). Bielefeld, Germany: Transcript-Verlag.

15 Basting (2006), p. 17.

16 Bungay, H., & Clift, S. (2010). Arts on prescription: A review of practice in the UK. *Perspectives in Public Health, 130*(6), 277–281.

17 Jensen, A., Stickley, T., Torrissen, W., & Stigmar, K. (2016). Arts on prescription in Scandinavia: A review of current practice and future possibilities. *Perspectives in Public Health, 137*(5), 268–274.

18 www.nccata.org

19 There are many types of validity and reliability, but in the simplest terms, validity means an instrument (like a questionnaire or test) has been shown to actually measure what it claims to measure, and reliability means that if you use the instrument several times, you should get similar results. For example, an unreliable bathroom scale will measure your weight in the morning as 130 pounds but in the evening at 150. That bathroom scale may be a valid (though unreliable) measure of your weight, but it is not a valid measure of your height.

20 One example comes from a study that attempted to determine whether a group participating in TimeSlips creative storytelling differed from a control group on mood and behavior as well as psychotropic medication use. They only had 10 participants in each group and found no differences between them. The authors suggested that with more participants and a longer study period, statistically significant differences might have been found: Houser, W. S., George, D. R., & Chinchilli, V. M. (2014). Impact of TimeSlips creative expression program on behavioral symptoms and psychotropic medication use in persons with dementia in long-term care: A cluster-randomized pilot study. *American Journal of Geriatric Psychiatry, 22,* 337–340.

21 One study even compared nine quantitative rating scales of agitation and anxiety to determine the best one to evaluate possible changes in residents participating in regular TimeSlips creative storytelling: Sullivan, E. L., Sillup, G. P., & Klimberg, R. K. (2014). TimeSlips—Comparing agitation and anxiety rating scales to evaluate the benefit of non-pharmacologic creative sessions in nursing home patients with dementia. *Open Journal of Nursing, 4,* 451–464.

22 The QoL-AD scale (Quality of Life—Alzheimer's Disease) has been translated into many languages and used in more than two thousand studies since being published in 2002: Logsdon, R., Gibbons, L. E., McCurry, S. M., & Teri, L. (2002). Assessing quality of life in older adults with cognitive impairment. *Psychosomatic Medicine, 64,* 510–519.

23 De Medeiros, K., & Basting, A. (2013). "Shall I compare thee to a dose of donepezil?": Cultural arts interventions in dementia care research. *The Gerontologist, 43,* 344–353.

24 Beard, R. (2011). Art therapies and dementia care: A systematic review. *Dementia, 11,* 633–656.

25 Camic, P. M., Crutch, S. J., Murphy, C., Firth, N. C., Harding, E., Harrison, C. R., et al. (2018). Conceptualising and understanding artistic creativity in the dementias: Interdisciplinary approaches to research and practise. *Frontiers in Psychology, 9,* 1–12. (p. 9)

26 Camic et al., p. 10.

27 Windle, G., Joling, K. J., Howson-Griffiths, T., Woods, B., Jones, C. H., van de Ven, P. H., et al. (2018). The impact of a visual arts program on quality of life, communication, and well-being of people living with dementia: A mixed-methods longitudinal investigation. *International Psychogeriatrics, 30,* 409–423. (p. 419)

28 Readers interested in studying this research further can consult the following articles whose titles usually are descriptive enough to indicate the focus of the investigations:

Bahlke, L. A., Pericolosi, S., & Lehman, M. E. (2010). Use of TimeSlips to improve communication in persons with moderate-late stage dementia. *Journal of Aging, Humanities, and the Arts, 4,* 390–405.

Chen, H-Y., Li, J., Wei, Y-P., Chen, P., & Li, H. (2016). Effects of TimeSlips on Cornell Scale for Depression in Dementia scores of senile dementia patients. *International Journal of Nursing Sciences, 3*(1), 35–38.

Fritsch, T., Kwak, J., Grant, S., Lang, J., Montgomery, R. R., & Basting, A. D. (2009). Impact of TimeSlips, a creative expression intervention program, on nursing home residents with dementia and their caregivers. *The Gerontologist, 49,* 117–126.

George, D. R., & Houser, W. S. (2014). "I'm a storyteller!": Exploring the benefits of TimeSlips creative expression program at a nursing home. *American Journal of Alzheimer's Disease and Other Dementias, 29,* 678–684.

George, D. R., Stuckey, H. L., Dillon, C. F., & Whitehead, M. M. (2011). Impact of participation in TimeSlips, a creative group-based storytelling program, on medical student attitudes toward persons with dementia: A qualitative study. *The Gerontologist, 51,* 699–713.

George, D. R., Stuckey, H. L., & Whitehead, M. M. (2014). How a creative storytelling intervention can improve medical student attitude towards persons with dementia: A mixed methods study. *Dementia, 13,* 318–329.

George, D. R., Yang, C., Stuckey, H. L., & Whitehead, M. M. (2012). Evaluating an arts-based intervention to improve medical student attitudes toward persons with dementia using the Dementia Attitudes Scale. *Journal of the American Geriatrics Society, 60,* 1583–1585.

Loizeau, A., Kündig, Y., & Oppikofer, S. (2015). "Awakened Art Stories"—Rediscovering pictures by persons living with dementia utilizing TimeSlips: A pilot study. *Geriatric Mental Health Care, 3,* 13–20.

Phillips, L. J., Reid-Arndt, S. A., & Pak, Y. (2010). Effects of a creative expression intervention on emotions, communication, and quality of life in persons with dementia. *Nursing Research, 59,* 417–425.

Swinnen, A., & de Medeiros, K. (2018). "Play" and people living with dementia: A humanities-based inquiry of TimeSlips and the Alzheimer's Poetry Project. *The Gerontologist, 58,* 261–269.

Vigliotti, A. A., Chinchilli, V. M., & George, D. R. (2017). Enhancing quality of life and caregiver interactions for persons with dementia using TimeSlips group storytelling: A 6-month longitudinal study. *American Journal of Geriatric Psychiatry, 26*(4), 507–508.

Chapter 10

Spiritual Connections

British poet and teacher John Killick once overheard the following conversation at an adult day center. Maria, a visiting musician, had just played a Bach piece and was talking with Bob, a participant at the center.

> Bob: You touch the very, the little strings in the center of my heart. What do you think of that now?
>
> Maria: I touch the strings in the center of your heart? Is that how you feel when you listen to music?
>
> Bob: Oh yes, oh yes I do, yes. It's something you can't explain. That's the way it is. There's something in you, like, I suppose mental as well as naturally, and I don't know, you can't explain it, that's the way it is.[1]

Bob is saying that he experiences "something more" when he hears the music. I use that phrase "something more" deliberately. It comes from the work of William James, the first American to write a psychology text and the author of *The Varieties of Religious Experience*, his book on the psychology of religion. James said that people have an inchoate sense that there is "something more" to this life and world beyond material existence.[2] Like Bob, they may not be able to explain it, but they know that it touches the "little strings" in their hearts. Some call it spirituality. James thought of it as what people seek from religion.

In the 1990s, a few gerontologists realized that their usual measures of what contributes to elders' well-being were failing to capture something important—something their data on physical health, financial security, and social connections could not account for. In other words, there was "something more" not included in their metrics. This motivated some researchers to study older adults' sense of spirituality and their religious beliefs and practices. In general, this research showed significant, positive correlations of measures of spirituality and religiousness with various physical and mental health outcomes for elders. Of course, most of these studies were not able to prove that spirituality or religiousness *caused* better physical health (for example, less hypertension and heart disease) and lower levels of loneliness, depression, and anxiety.[3] However, after about two decades of research, social scientists seemed willing to accept that positive outcomes accrued to older people who welcomed "something more" into their lives.

Nearly all these researchers began their books and papers by wrestling with definitions of religion and spirituality.[4] Although the two constructs were once securely fused, by the end of the twentieth century they had split apart, with the identity of being "spiritual but not religious" gaining popularity. Arguments about definitions often hinged on whether spirituality necessarily included a transcendent being beyond the self or whether it reflected human qualities not dependent upon religious beliefs and practices.

After quoting the exchange between Bob and Maria, Killick offered a definition of spirituality reflecting the contemporary splitting of religion and spirituality. He called spirituality

> the search for that which gives zest, energy, meaning and identity to a person's life, in relation to other people, and to the wider world. Spirituality can be experienced in feelings of awe or wonder, those moments of life which take you beyond the mundane into a sacred place.[5]

Bob's expression of his feelings of awe and wonder when he heard Maria play the piece by Bach reveals how art has the potential to transform the mundane into the numinous.

Of course, some might say that listening to the music of Bach is an obvious example of the intertwining of art and spirituality. However, I have felt this connection in less obvious situations such as observing people living with dementia engage with the arts. For example, when I witnessed the joy of the nursing-home residents, staff, and family members described in the previous chapter as they sang and danced in *Wendy's Neverland*, it felt like a transcendent moment—a spiritual moment—to me. My usual assumptions about life in a rural, Medicaid-dependent nursing home fell away, replaced with a deep sense of connection with these people I had never met and would never see again. Yet, the memory of that experience— especially of the moments when I sang "I'll Fly Away" with the woman using a wheelchair—is like a jewel, sparkling and clear, just like memories I have of experiences usually associated with the emotion of awe, such as when I held our newborn child or when I witness sunshine break through storm clouds over a lake.

I also experience awe when I am with a person living with dementia who patiently sculpts with clay, contributes a wise detail to an unfolding story, or meditatively constructs complex arrays of stones and leaves. Awe, according to psychologists, results from perceptions of vastness that force us to change our assumptions about what we are experiencing.[6] We ordinarily associate awe with moments such as when we view a sunset from the edge of the Grand Canyon, moments when we suddenly have to revise our notions of our own stature and importance. The awe felt when interacting openly and authentically with a person living with dementia can come from realizing the vastness of a human life built up layer by layer over decades, much of which may now be hidden. However, when we see a person who rarely speaks mouth the words to a song, or when a person slumped in a wheelchair picks up a brush and paints a bright yellow flower, we find ourselves forced to alter our assumptions about dementia and people living with the condition.

In addition to my awe in observing the creative expression of people living with dementia, I am awed by the courage and strength of care partners who accompany their loved ones to memory cafés or to our chorus practices, often on frigid, snowy Wisconsin winter days. They relax, greet friends, and set aside the stresses of caregiving for a few hours. I am also awed by the resilience of poorly paid nursing-home aides who consistently treat residents with compassion. To say this another way, many of my interactions with people living with dementia remind me of what Viktor Frankl called the "defiant power of the human spirit."[7] Although the word "defiant" carries connotations of fighting or stubborn resistance, Frankl meant simply that human beings persist; despite mounting losses and daily tribulations, humans generally persist in trying to make life as good as possible.

Frankl, a Viennese psychoanalyst imprisoned in four Nazi concentration camps, spoke about spirituality as the search for meaning and called this the primary motivational force for human beings.[8] He told the story of the origins of these ideas in his well-known book *Man's Search for Meaning*. Later, he wrote that religions guide people in their "search for ultimate meaning."[9] Although some Holocaust scholars now debate the significance of his work, it has influenced many people interested in the role of religion and spirituality in older people's lives, because so much about old age, particularly in Western cultures, seems to have been stripped of meaning.[10]

A Relational Model of Spirituality

Elizabeth MacKinlay, an Anglican priest and registered nurse in Australia who earned a PhD with a thesis on the spiritual dimension of aging, frequently travels worldwide giving talks about her work. She addresses the loss of meaning for elders, including those living with dementia, in her research, in her many books, and at the international conferences on aging and spirituality she has organized. Influenced by her studies of Frankl's writings, as well as her clinical practice in residential care communities, she has developed a model illustrating four ways spirituality is mediated in human beings. She has also coauthored articles with Christine Bryden (introduced in Chapters 4 and 5), who came to her after being diagnosed with a type of dementia. Bryden sought a spiritual guide for journeying through the strange land of dementia, a role MacKinlay felt initially reluctant to undertake. Together, they sought understanding about how people can find meaning amidst the day-to-day challenges of memory loss and other expressions of dementia.[11] MacKinlay described her journey with Bryden as one of her "most significant life experiences."[12]

In interviews with people living with dementia, and in group discussions using her technique of "spiritual reminiscence,"[13] MacKinlay heard elders describe the sources of deepest meaning in their lives. MacKinlay's spiritual reminiscence method uses guided discussions about happy and sad times in their lives, feelings about formal and informal spiritual and religious practices, what they look forward to in their remaining years, and how others can offer meaningful assistance to them.

By far the most commonly named source of meaning by the elders in MacKinlay's groups came from human relationships. MacKinlay saw these relationships as expressing spirituality. These were not casual relationships, but rather meaningful connections with others in what MacKinlay viewed as a sacred space. As MacKinlay learned from Bryden and the very elderly people in her spiritual reminiscence groups, some people also experience a deep connection with God, understood by Christians as triune (consisting of Creator, Christ, and Spirit). According to Christian theology, the relationship of Trinity is woven together with an all-encompassing love that is offered to all human beings. For Bryden, this is an essential. In an essay describing her spiritual journey, she wrote:

> As the body of Christ, His church, we are in fellowship with each other and with God. I can be held in this relationship and be part of our corporate community with the divine. This relationship is one of divine love, which is unconditional. Such love does not need me to behave normally or consistently; it does not need me to know who you are or even who I am. We bear one another in love.[14]

A spiritual sense of ultimate meaning can also be mediated through relationships with the natural environment, an experience often described as sacred by persons who may or may not introduce a transcendent being into their ideas about spirituality. A moving example of this comes from a story told by Eileen Shamy, a British Methodist pastor who wrote one of the first books about ministry with people having dementia. She once asked the daughters of a woman with dementia what had nourished her spirit as she coped with the trials of living in England during World War II. They recalled that she often told them how she had walked in a park with large, old trees every day during the War. She had said, "The trees gave me their strength." A few days after Shamy's conversation with her daughters, aides at her nursing home wrapped her in a warm blanket and wheeled her to a nearby park. That evening, she was not her usual, restless, anxious self. Rather, she snuggled into her bed and told her nurse, "I tasted the sky; God held me up."[15] These were probably her last words; she died peacefully a week later. This story of an old woman experiencing a spiritual connection with the environment will feel familiar to people who have taken the time to sit quietly with a person living with dementia, sharing a moment of feeling the breeze, looking at a flower garden, hearing birdsong, and experiencing other ordinary but profoundly meaningful encounters with the natural world.

In addition to meaningful connections with humans and with God, and with the natural world, MacKinlay believes that a third way of mediating the spiritual comes from experiencing the arts in their many forms. She describes how these moments can elicit awe when people—including those who are deeply forgetful—connect with music, visual art, poetry, drama, dance, and other artistic expressions. As I mentioned earlier, this awe can also be felt by people observing persons living with dementia express themselves through creativity. Earlier in the dementia process, creative expression may be an outgrowth of a lifetime of pursuing some form of art; later in the progression, a guide may be needed. Fortunately, more artists are being trained to work with people living with dementia, and art museums are offering programs for them and their care partners to create art and imaginatively respond to works of art. These programs mediate spirituality not only through the art form but also through the relationships of people with the artists leading the programs.

The fourth component of MacKinlay's model of spirituality is religion. She does not view religion as isolated from spirituality, although, of course, many people do experience such a division as a result of their negative and sometimes painful experiences of religious traditions. Religious rules and hierarchical structures can prevent them from feeling meaningful spiritual connections with the divine, other people, the natural world, or even the arts (since some religious groups regard the arts as threatening to their worldview). For MacKinlay, religion offers symbols, stories, rituals, and practices such as prayer and meditation that gather together all of the other ways in which spirituality is mediated. She recognizes and respects the diversity of religious faiths and relates her observations of religious practices in care communities for Jews, Buddhists, Muslims, and

Hindus, as well as her own tradition of Christianity. For example, when visiting a small group home in Japan, she saw how staff members enabled a woman who could no longer speak or walk to worship at her Buddhist altar twice a day. This act signified a spiritual connection not only as a religious practice but also because it involved the care of another human being supporting that religious practice.

MacKinlay's four-part model describing spirituality represents her attempt to uncover sources of Frankl's "defiant power of the human spirit"—that resilience that keeps us striving to be useful, positive, and loving. Dementia does not rob people of their ability to express this power, though sometimes it can be quite subtle, as in the squeeze of a hand or a flickering smile.

Before elaborating on MacKinlay's last point about religious practices having developed through centuries of people coming together in communities—which now sometimes identify as dementia-friendly faith communities—a brief, light-touch detour into theology is called for. After all, it is easy and sometimes facile to toss around references to the "human spirit" and to lift up poignant examples of its defiant qualities in people living with dementia. But what do we really mean?

Theological Reflections on the Human Spirit

Theologians from many faith traditions have repeatedly upheld the ideal of the rational human as possessing all of one's cognitive faculties as well as the ability to reflect at length on divinity and its relation to humanity—an ideal that excludes most people living with dementia. Recently, however, a few theologians have discovered that consideration of the many challenges presented by dementia offers a pathway into engagement with critical theological issues. In fact, Peter Kevern, a British theologian, has urged that when people first receive a dementia diagnosis they should consult with a spiritual adviser who can walk with them through the treacherous terrain of questions such as "Why did God let this happen to me?" and "What is the point of living any longer?" Kevern argues that these conversations are just as important early in the dementia journey as are consultations with medical professionals, attorneys, and financial counselors.[16]

John Swinton is a Scottish theologian and former psychiatric nurse in a ward for people with advanced dementia. Today he is one of the leading theologians writing about dementia. In his book *Dementia: Living in the Memories of God*, Swinton calls dementia a cultural as well as a biological disease because of the way culture afflicts people having dementia symptoms with negative stereotypes and social exclusion. Swinton finds in the Christian story a counter-story that radically rewrites the culturally accepted biomedical stories of terrifying decline. The story he wants to tell is grounded not only in what he calls the "big stories" of the Bible—the Exodus, the Cross, redemption—but also in the smaller stories of human life, including those involving people who are often excluded from the faith communities that supposedly are open to all believers (though many have strict ideas about who can be called a believer).[17]

Swinton asserts that the only way to understand the human spirit is to start by "understanding who God is and where human beings stand in relation to God."[18] Swinton begins what he calls his exercise in theological anthropology by talking about human contingency and dependency: human beings are loved and valued by God through all of life's joys and sufferings, including those wrought by dementia. Coinciding with much important work being done today by scholars in fields other than theology,[19] Swinton asserts that we cannot fully understand the experience of dementia without acknowledging the fact that "human beings are embodied creatures."[20] The contingency of human life is wound up in embodiment, which Swinton believes is expressed in the Hebrew Bible's story of creation. The book of Genesis tells the story of humans formed of dust and becoming living beings by receiving the breath of God, the *nephesh*. In this view, bodies are holy ground, so that even the smallest acts of care, such as washing a face, massaging lotion into hands, or rubbing feet, reflect "divine love for dependent human beings."[21] For Swinton, the human spirit is animated by the *nephesh*.

Rabbi Dayle Friedman (mentioned in Chapter 6) also refers to the Hebrew Biblical creation story in order to reflect theologically on dementia. She regards the *tzelem*, the divine spark in humans, as remaining in all persons regardless of the changes occurring in the brain that produce the symptoms that disturb them and the people who love and care for them. Friedman believes it is the role of all who give care—both the unpaid care of family members and friends, and the care of paid persons—to seek the *tzelem* in people living with dementia. By doing this, they can discover that "in the person who is disoriented, who is regressed, or even unresponsive, somehow the image of God resides."[22]

Dementia has been called the "theological disease"[23] because it elicits profound questions for many people about meaning, suffering, and human nature itself. Although a theologian might engage with these questions from a strictly academic perspective, MacKinlay, Swinton, and Friedman gift their readers with a different approach. In addition to their roles in academia, all have for many years worked as chaplains serving communities of people living with dementia and other disabilities. They have witnessed the fear and confusion when a diagnosis is first delivered, accompanied people and their care partners in the progression of symptoms, and ministered to individuals in dementia's very late stages. They have led religious services in care communities where some individuals show little response to the worship experience. In other words, their theological engagement with dementia is grounded in a personal history of relationships in which they have sought the *tzelem*.

For Swinton and Friedman, the defiant power of the human spirit described by Frankl comes from the animating breath of God. This affirmation is nurtured and expressed through communal engagement with religious rituals when the community gathers in a place Swinton describes as being "where the implications of the *nephesh* that inspires and binds human beings together are recognized and named and its Giver worshipped."[24] Similarly, Friedman offers many examples of how Jewish rituals, songs, and celebrations of holy days "empower individuals to live in sacred time."[25] An implication of the work of Friedman, Swinton, and others who engage with the theological questions of meaning, suffering, and humanity raised by dementia is that faith communities declaring themselves to be dementia friendly are radically different from secular social organizations that welcome people living with dementia.[26] Memory cafés offer delightful, friendly experiences and may elicit feelings of spiritual connection among those who attend them, but they are not predicated on shared convictions and practices focused on human relationships with the sacred.

Dementia-Friendly and Inclusive Faith Communities

A few years ago, I conducted interviews with pastors to learn how they responded to people in their congregations who were living with dementia. I heard a variety of responses. One pastor of a large evangelical congregation told me that most of the members are in their 30s and 40s and "are more concerned with their kids."[27] He concluded this after offering an adult class on "dealing with parents in the golden years." He said it "wasn't a hot topic" and went on to tell me that he did not think people were wrestling with theological questions involving aging and dementia because they do not have "a big vision of the future." Another pastor of a similar congregation told me that his church has a group called the "nifty fifty" who do "a lot of social things," but he thinks "we are always going to be a young person's church." He described his church as attracting between 2,500 and 3,000 people on a weekend, but he knew of only one care partner in the whole congregation. As the interview ended, I suggested that perhaps some of the young and middle-aged people attending his church have parents and grandparents living with dementia. He paused a long time and then said, "My sister and brother and I are starting to run into that with my dad."

I got a very different response from a woman pastoring with a more traditional faith community where she estimated that two thirds of the Christian congregation ranges in age from the 40s through the 60s, with the other third split between older people and younger people. She firmly stated her belief that the church has a role to be prophetic to the culture by speaking out about inclusion of people with memory loss. She told me several stories about how her congregation lived this idea. For example, she described the challenge of working with a woman diagnosed with the early stage of dementia who chaired their stewardship committee (the group in charge of collecting financial commitments from members). She said, "It is an act of mercy that she is still in that position. We all know what's going on, and we work around it. She really loves doing this; I just couldn't tell her she had to resign." The downside of this mercy, said the pastor, was that the committee was not working to its fullest potential. The pastor believed that the issue could be handled, since the woman only had a year left of her six-year term. She told me other stories centered on the importance of sharing meals at her church and the ways they find roles for people with dementia to continue helping in the church kitchen.

At the end of my interview with her, this pastor told me a poignant story. She was taking communion to someone with Alzheimer's disease whose daughter asked why she was bothering to do this. She replied that this was about God, not her mother's memory. She went on to say, "I'll be giving communion to someone completely out of it, and I'll give the bread and wine. As soon as I start to say the Lord's Prayer, they are saying it right with me word for word. You see the light in their eyes. I can't explain it, but there's something there. Theologically, we need to understand that we are embodied souls." In other words, this pastor is able to see the *tzelem*, the divine spark. Similar to Swinton, this pastor said that even in people with advanced dementia, "God is still present in the person."

In recent years, a number of publications have offered guidance for faith communities seeking to include and serve people living with dementia. Before reviewing their recommendations, we need to pause to ask whether this intention actually matters in a time when fewer people of any age are engaged with these communities, especially in Europe, the United Kingdom, and the United States. One answer comes from an abundant literature on religion, spirituality, and aging documenting that elders today tend to engage in both private and public religious practices at a far higher rate than younger persons.[28]

Like the first two pastors whose interviews I described, some congregations deliberately shape their worship style, educational offerings, and social gatherings to attract young adults and their families. In other, more traditional, faith communities such as the one served by the pastor in the last interview, the marks of age can easily be seen in the majority of congregants. This observation, and the demographic literature on religiousness, should not, however, produce the specious assumption that most older people are religious. After over 40 years studying religion and aging in the UK and Europe, British psychologist Peter Coleman and his colleagues concluded that although many older people do remain faithful to their original religious identity and convictions, others have left their faith communities and rejected the authority of religious teachings. The researchers also noted an increasing influence of "Eastern spirituality and a more personalized approach to prayer and conception of God."[29] The implications for people living with dementia of these diverse responses to the changing religious landscape worldwide have not been adequately investigated. However, there is considerable evidence that those who retain their traditional religious faith, practices, and community affiliations find sustenance that supports their ability to cope, hold on to hope, and continue to find meaning in their lives.[30]

In her chapter in the book about dementia-friendly communities in Germany, Verena Rothe (mentioned in Chapters 7 and 9) observed that religious congregations "offer some good indicators for seeing and understanding what is important in a dementia-friendly community."[31] She said this not only because they sometimes have special services for people living with dementia and provide pastoral care for individuals and families but also because they offer a structure for thinking about dementia similar to what Swinton and Friedman described.

The rapidly spreading dementia-friendly and inclusive movement has recognized the services and care offered by faith communities, though without acknowledging the theology underpinning them. For example, the Dementia Friendly America (DFA) organization has a page on its website devoted to faith communities. Using its structure of "prepare, learn, respond," DFA recommends educating faith communities about signs of dementia, the importance of early diagnosis, and local services that help people living with dementia. It offers suggestions about communication strategies and practical advice, such as the importance of having everyone wear nametags. Ideas about engaging with people having dementia and care partners range from offering shorter, simpler services to home visits that "create spiritual connections and maximize interaction through familiar prayer or scripture or traditional hymns."[32]

A booklet written by Baptist minister Gaynor Hammond, and produced in England by a collaboration of religious groups, goes further than the DFA guide. (The DFA guide also addresses banks, law offices, libraries, and hospitals.) Hammond begins by boldly stating that becoming a dementia-friendly and inclusive congregation involves more than installing ramps, hearing loops (sound systems for people using hearing aids), and "comfy seats." Also, personal interactions need to go beyond "offering a friendly welcome at the door." Although these accommodations are important, being a dementia-friendly and inclusive church is about looking for ways in which those who have dementia, along with their families and friends, can feel they are completely included as valued members of the congregation. It is about accepting and valuing people regardless of cognitive abilities and being open to what people with dementia have to offer.[33]

Hammond provides practical suggestions about creating meaningful worship for people who have dementia, whether with the whole congregation, as a shorter service for people with dementia and care partners, in a care community, or in people's homes. She also gives examples of how spiritual needs change with dementia progression and offers ideas about compassionately responding to challenges faced by people in the early, middle, and late stages of dementia.

Regardless of where people are in the progression of dementia, they may encounter unfriendliness in faith communities. For example, unlike the response of the pastor of the traditional congregation who told me about the stewardship chairman with dementia who was accommodated, Hammond relates a story about a woman who had faithfully served on her church's refreshments team but could no longer bake the lovely cakes she used to bring on Sundays. One Sunday, the team surprised her with a bouquet of flowers, thanked her for her service, and told her it was time for her to be waited on by them. This sudden "firing" was an emotional blow, making her feel rejected and unappreciated. In another example of unfriendliness, Hammond tells the story of Betty, a faithful member of a church, now living in a nursing home. Diagnosed with dementia, Betty nevertheless wanted to visit with friends who regularly gathered at her church for coffee once a week. Her daughter, Sally, agreed to take her to the coffee gathering, but after greeting her with hugs, no one tried to engage Betty in conversation. Sally said that she saw her mother "shrink into herself," and on the way home Betty plaintively commented, "No one wanted to talk to me, did they?"[34]

The story of Betty and Sally is far too common. Faith communities are human organizations, subject to human flaws and prejudices. Nevertheless, they have rich resources to offer people journeying into dementia along with their care partners. Researchers have documented care partners' views about the effectiveness of spiritual coping practices such as prayer and meditation, as well as attendance at religious services.[35] They have also interviewed people living with dementia and concluded that religious identities offer strength and hope, the ability to maintain a positive attitude, contentment, and meaningful connections with other persons.[36]

In addition to directly ministering with care partners and their loved ones with dementia, faith communities that embrace the mission of being dementia friendly need to begin by being dementia inclusive. They should ask people living with dementia what they want from their faith communities and the role they wish to play, even as the dementia progresses. Otherwise, if they do not consult with the people most affected by dementia, they are failing to honor the people they claim to be serving. Based on the stated needs and desires of people living with dementia, this service could include

- advocating for improvements in respite care, adult day services, and other programs to serve families dealing with dementia

- enlarging their view of mission to include support for establishing memory cafés and other social programs in their cities and towns (perhaps using their own classrooms and meeting spaces)

- addressing transportation challenges in order to alleviate loneliness among people living with dementia

- training people to be regular visitors for those with dementia and their care partners

- encouraging clergy to become better educated about ministry with people having dementia[37]

- urging long-term care organizations to hire chaplains

- honoring the work of certified nursing assistants, whose daily tasks are infused with opportunities for providing spiritually meaningful connections.

Faith Communities and Long-Term Care

A few years ago I worked with some talented college students who developed a six-week plan to bring arts programming into a skilled nursing home that mostly served Medicaid-supported residents. Because the nursing home was next door to a large church, we assumed that the church would be a logical place to recruit volunteers to help with the arts program. We contacted the pastor several times, but he told us that he was unable to generate any enthusiasm for participating in our program. We offered to come to the church to talk about what we planned to do, but we were rebuffed. Finally, we approached another congregation several miles away and enlisted the help of three energetic women who contributed much to the creative-engagement activities and reported that they gained much in doing so. I still think, based on my experience working with many faith communities, that we might have recruited similarly enthusiastic people from the original church we contacted if we had received more support from the pastor, who appeared to see no value in arts activities for nursing-home residents living with dementia.

I also know, from being married to a pastor for 50 years, that leading a congregation is a highly demanding, time-consuming job, with plenty of rewards and multiple sources of frustration. Regarding ministry with elders, clergy receive little training in seminary about aging, and even less about dementia. In his appraisal of this situation, Malcolm Goldsmith, a Scottish Episcopalian vicar and research fellow at the Dementia Services Development Centre at Stirling University, stated that in his experience "most clergy are good people and well-meaning." However, he went on to say that "like most of the population they are generally ignorant about dementia and find it confusing and unnerving when they are asked to minister to people with dementia and their families."[38] This clergy discomfort may drive away congregational members living with dementia who end up feeling invisible and forgotten.

For over a decade, beginning in 1994, several colleagues and I tried to remediate this situation through the curriculum we developed for the Gerontological Pastoral Care Institute (GPCI), which was organized by the Center on Aging, Religion, and Spirituality (CARS) at Luther Seminary in St. Paul, Minnesota. I believe that I learned more from the pastors and chaplains participating in the program than they learned from me. I heard their stories about not having time to visit parishioners living in long-term-care communities. They told me about not knowing what to say or how to interact with people living with advanced dementia. Often they realized that bringing their lengthy, complex Sunday sermon to preach again on Wednesday afternoon at the nursing home was not appropriate, but they did not know what else they could do. No helpful toolkits, pamphlets, or brochures had been developed for dementia-friendly faith communities or even age-friendly faith communities. To begin to address this, my colleagues and I edited a handbook on religion, spirituality, and aging published in 1995. However, several years later, we realized that dementia was hardly mentioned in the handbook.[39] We corrected that omission in the second volume, which contained five chapters specifically about dementia along with other chapters that included some mention of people living with dementia.[40]

Almost half of the participants in the GPCI program came from the world of nursing-home chaplaincy. They often commented on what Debbie Everett, a Canadian chaplain, has described as the hierarchy of chaplaincy prestige: hospital chaplains are ranked as having the highest status, military and prison chaplains are ranked somewhere in the middle, and nursing-home chaplains are ranked at the bottom of the status hierarchy.[41] Ageism and dementism shaped how other people responded to the chaplains' professional commitments. These other people assumed, for example, that the chaplains could not succeed as parish clergy so they "escaped" to nursing homes where few skills seemed to be needed to minister with elders, especially those having dementia. Like Everett, chaplains often heard comments about how they were "wasting time" trying to minister to residents with dementia. But also, like Everett, they told me about the surprising paradox woven through this ministry: when visiting with and serving residents living with advanced dementia, the chaplains were freed from their "intellectual theological boxes" and were introduced "to a God who is also dancing and laughing in the bizarre places where chaos reigns."[42]

In 1998, after I attended the Pioneer Network conference in Oshkosh, Wisconsin, and learned about Tom Kitwood's book *Dementia Reconsidered*, I sent a letter to the GPCI chaplains asking them to write me letters with descriptions of how they cared for residents' grief. I asked this because the CCRC that sponsored the Oshkosh conference was moving to a new model of care through an architectural transformation creating small households in one large building with 11 residents each; a group of four households was called a neighborhood. I saw this as a vast improvement over the hospital-like design of so many nursing homes built in the 1950s and 60s, but I wondered about the relational issues in these new settings. If a nursing home is creating a "household" or a "neighborhood," does this not imply that residents will get to know one another, and if so, what happens when a fellow resident dies?

I received many poignant replies from the chaplains, who told me how they saw their roles as community keepers. One chaplain shared a story that will be familiar to anyone who has worked in a long-term care residence. She described a loud and belligerent man who disturbed others. One woman who lived there was able to let him be; another tried to calm him. When the man was dying, the chaplain sensed that the two women knew something was happening: "They would hover in the hall area near his door, walking hand in hand, making only little short walks before returning and walking past the door again." She told them that the man was very sick and dying. One of the women, a Catholic who rarely spoke, managed to say, "Is he good?" After the man died, the chaplain returned to the unit, where she found the women still pacing near the doorway of the man's room. "I just put my arm around them, and we walked into the bare, empty room with the bed stripped of its coverings, and we stood there." Having known that words would probably be inadequate, she wrote that "to just enter the empty room seemed to be the best pastoral response, along with my presence with them, my arm around them."

Chaplains related other stories like this. For instance, one of my correspondents told me about residents being disturbed by frequent staff changes. They would become emotionally attached to a nursing assistant, only to have that person disappear. The chaplain emphasized the need to acknowledge these feelings, for example through what she called a "reflective service" that recognized and dealt with their grief over the loss of so many people and things in their lives. She concluded her letter by saying that she often uses poetry, music, and puppet plays when creating rituals for residents, because "imagination and creativity can relate to the situation and circumstances of the loss or transition."

Most long-term care residences do not employ chaplains. So who will address this kind of grief for the majority of persons in long-term care facilities? Who will employ that "imagination and creativity" to connect with people who have lost language and often seem out of touch with their environment? Sometimes a residence employs a "lifestyle coordinator" or activities director, but will they have time to comfort grieving residents? In my experience, this role often falls to the certified nursing assistant (CNA). Although places where CNAs work may look fancy on the outside and charge high monthly rates for care, hourly pay for CNAs remains low, and often they have little to no training in caring for people living with dementia. According to the US Bureau of Labor Statistics, in 2018 the median annual pay for a CNA was $28,530.[43] This is only $2,780 above the 2019 US poverty guideline for a family of four.[44]

In his 2004 book *In a Strange Land: People with Dementia and the Local Church*, Malcolm Goldsmith included a talk he gave to CNAs at a nursing home outside of Sydney, Australia. After reflecting on how hard their jobs are, he told them:

> You are part of that great mass of men and women who catch occasional glimpses of glory, recognize moments of grace, and for most of the time get on with your working and your living.[45]

In other words, Goldsmith was talking about how CNAs can witness the *tzelem* in a resident's smile, feel it in a squeeze of a hand, and hear it in the residents' sighs of contentment when the CNA gently cares for their embodied selves. The human spirits of the residents in their care reflect the first breath—the *nephesh*. Sometimes, that breath is all the resident has to give. Helping CNAs to see their routine tasks as expressions of spirituality—of creating meaningful connections with others, the arts, nature, and religious practices—can add meaning, purpose, and hope to their work. Faith communities that embrace a mission of bringing more justice to the world of dementia care could raise their voices to support better pay, training, and respect for CNAs.

Spiritual Accompaniment

In Chapter 6, when describing Grace's commitment to Suzy, I referred to Rabbi Friedman's writing about spiritual accompaniment—*livui ruchani*. This is a role many people could undertake in a dementia-friendly and inclusive faith community. Clergy do this (or should do this) with people living with dementia. Chaplains working in long-term-care communities do this every day, along with many of the CNAs and other staff caring for the residents (although the work of staff members may not be cast in this light, since all too often it is viewed only as checking tasks off a long list). Friends like Grace do this. Members of faith communities can also be encouraged to embrace this role, and many already do this by being a deacon or friendly visitor. A commitment to offer spiritual accompaniment to a person living with dementia could give care partners much-needed respite. It could also offer hope in the form of a promise that neither the person living with dementia nor the care partner will be abandoned as the symptoms worsen.

As the dementia progresses, having conversations with the person with dementia about the spiritual challenges they may face might no longer be possible. At that point, other meaningful ways of connecting with the person will need to be substituted. These will often involve some form of the arts. Shared time together could take the form of reciting a poem in a call-and-response manner, moving rhythmically to music, playing a person's favorite song on a ukulele, making up a story about an amusing photograph, and myriad other experiences that can touch the strings in the center of a person's heart just like Maria's playing of the Bach piece touched Bob.

This is not a case of *doing for* another person, but of *doing with* and *being with*. This kind of meaningful connection—which can be understood as spiritual regardless of a person's religiousness—offers many rewards. People living with dementia, including in the last stages, have much to offer those who accompany them in these meaningful ways. After all, consider that many people (including persons experiencing the early stage of dementia) pay a lot of money to go to workshops to learn mindfulness techniques. They could also learn how to be fully present in the moment by spending time with an individual living with the middle or later stages of dementia. Each encounter will be different, and some visits will feel decidedly unspiritual and not at all peaceful. However, with practice, patience, and careful observation of what brings joy and meaning to another person, it is possible to grasp the profound meaning of the *tzelem* and understand that the *nephesh* is something that can be shared.

Endnotes

1 Killick, J. (2004). Magic mirrors: What people with dementia show us about ourselves. In A. Jewell (Ed.), *Ageing, spirituality, and well-being* (pp. 143–152). New York, NY: Jessica Kingsley Publishers. (p. 147)

2 James, W. (1961). *The varieties of religious experience.* New York, NY: Collier Books. (p. 401) (Original work published 1901).

3 For a comprehensive survey of research on the relation of spirituality and religiousness with physical and mental health, see this handbook: Koenig, H. G., King, D. E., & Carson, V. B. (2012). *Handbook of religion and health* (2nd ed.). New York, NY: Oxford University Press.

4 One article by a psychologist cited 12 definitions of religion and 14 definitions of spirituality: Oman, D. (2013). Religion and spirituality: Evolving meanings and prototypes. In R. F. Paloutzian & C. L. Park (Eds.), *Handbook of the psychology of religion and spirituality* (2nd ed., pp. 23–47). New York, NY: Guilford Press.

5 Froggatt, A., & Moffitt, L. (1997). Spiritual needs and religious practice in dementia care. In M. Marshall (Ed.), *State of the art in dementia care.* London, UK: Centre for Policy on Ageing. Quoted in Killick, p. 149.

6 Keltner, D., & Haidt, J. (2003). Approaching awe, a moral, spiritual, and aesthetic emotion. *Cognition and Emotion, 17,* 297–314.

7 Frankl, V. (1967). *Psychotherapy and existentialism: Selected papers on logotherapy.* New York, NY: Washington Square Press. (p. 99)

8 Frankl, V. (1984). *Man's search for meaning.* New York, NY: Washington Square Press. (Original work published 1946)

9 Frankl, V. (1975). *The unconscious God.* New York, NY: Washington Square Press. (p. 13)

10 Kimble, M. A. (1995). Pastoral care. In M. A. Kimble, S. H. McFadden, J. W. Ellor, & J. J. Seeber (Eds.), *Aging, spirituality, and religion: A handbook* (pp. 131–147). Minneapolis, MN: Fortress Press.

11 Bryden, C., & MacKinlay, E. (2002). Dementia—A spiritual journey toward the divine: A personal view of dementia. In E. MacKinlay (Ed.), *Mental health and spirituality in later life* (pp. 69–75). New York, NY: The Haworth Pastoral Press.

12 MacKinlay, E. (2017). *The spiritual dimension of ageing.* Philadelphia, PA: Jessica Kingsley Publishers. (p. 331)

13 Trevitt, C., & MacKinlay, E. (2004). "Just because I can't remember...": Religiousness in older people with dementia. In E. MacKinlay (Ed.), *Spirituality of later life: On humor and despair* (pp. 109–121). New York, NY: Haworth Pastoral Press.

14 Bryden, C. (2016). A spiritual journey into the I-Thou relationship: A personal reflection on living with dementia. *Journal of Religion, Spirituality, and Aging, 28,* 7–14. (pp. 11–12)

15 Shamy, E. (2003). *A guide to the spiritual dimension of care for people with Alzheimer's disease and related dementia: More than body, brain, and breath.* London, UK: Jessica Kingsley Publishers. (p. 83)

16 Kevern, P. (2011). "I pray that I will not fall over the edge": What is left of faith after dementia? *Practical Theology, 4*(3), 283–294.

17 In an earlier book, Swinton addressed the ways faith communities fear and exclude people with serious mental-health problems such as schizophrenia: Swinton, J. (2000). *Resurrecting the person: Friendship and the care of people with mental health problems.* Nashville, TN: Abington Press.

18 Swinton, J. (2012). *Dementia: Living in the memories of God.* Grand Rapids, MI: William B. Eerdmans Publishing. (p. 160)

19 Since the 1990s, Pia Kontos has conducted research highlighting the embodied selfhood of people living with dementia. Recently, she has connected this work to a model of relational citizenship that emphasizes reciprocity between people living with dementia in long-term-care communities and their caregivers: Kontos, P., Miller, K-L., & Kontos, A. P. (2017). Relational citizenship: Supporting embodied selfhood and relationality in dementia care. *Sociology of Health & Illness, 39*, 182–198.

20 Swinton (2012), p. 165.

21 Swinton (2012), p. 171.

22 Friedman, D. A. (2008). *Jewish visions for aging: A professional guide for fostering wholeness.* Woodstock, VT: Jewish Lights Publishing. (p. 48)

23 Keck, D. (1996). *Forgetting whose we are: Alzheimer's disease and the love of God.* Nashville, TN: Abington Press.

24 Swinton (2012), p. 223.

25 Friedman, p. 51.

26 Unfortunately, I am less familiar with theological perspectives on dementia that are grounded in other faith traditions, such as Islam, Hinduism, and Buddhism. Peter Coleman and colleagues offered a perspective based on their studies of religious diversity among elders in the UK, with particular attention paid to Muslims. However, dementia was not their focal topic: Coleman, P. G., Begum, A, & Jaleel, S. (2011). Religious difference and age: The growing presence of other faiths. In P. G. Coleman, *Belief and ageing: Spiritual pathways in later life* (pp. 139–155). Portland, OR: Policy Press.

   A paper by Vance briefly outlined spiritual activities from these faith traditions that he believes can engage people living with dementia: Vance, D. E. (2004). Spiritual activities for adults with Alzheimer's disease: The cognitive components of dementia and religion. *Journal of Religion, Spirituality, and Aging, 17*(1/2), 109–130.

27 All the quotes from these interviews, and from the letters described later, are from studies that received approval from the Institutional Research Board at the university where I taught.

28 McFadden, S. H. (2015). Spirituality, religion, and aging: Clinical geropsychology and aging people's need for meaning. In P. A. Lichtenberg & B. T. Mast (Eds.), *APA handbook of clinical geropsychology* (Vol. 1, pp. 473–496). Washington, DC: American Psychological Association.

29 Coleman, P. G. (2011). The changing social context of belief in later life. In P. G. Coleman, *Belief and ageing: Spiritual pathways in later life* (pp. 11–33). Portland, OR: Policy Press.

30 Agli, O., Bailly, N., & Ferrand, C. (2015). Spirituality and religion in older adults with dementia: A systematic review. *International Psychogeriatrics, 27*, 715–725.

31 Rothe, V. (2017). People in the community living with dementia: The programme. In V. Rothe, G. Kruetzner, & R. Gronemeyer (Eds.), *Staying in life: Paving the way to dementia-friendly communities* (pp. 43–239). Bielefeld, Germany: Transcript-Verlag. (p. 71)

32 Dementia Friendly America. (2017). *Faith communities.* Washington, DC: Dementia Friendly America. Accessed on 8/15/19 at https://static1.squarespace.com/static/559c4229e4b0482682e8df9b/t/59aea8f59f8dce4ac7dfe77c/1504618741644/DFA-SectorGuide-Faith+8.9.17.pdf (p. 3)

33 Hammond, G. (2014). *Growing dementia-friendly churches.* Leeds, UK: Faith in Elderly People Leeds/Christian Council on Aging/Methodist Homes Association. (p. 6)

34 Hammond, p. 19.

35 Hebert, R. S., Dang, Q., & Sculz, R. (2007). Religious beliefs and practices are associated with better mental health in family caregivers of patients with dementia: Findings from the REACH study. *American Journal of Geriatric Psychiatry, 15*(4), 292–300.

36 Sullivan, S. C., & Beard, R. L. (2014). Faith and forgetfulness: The role of spiritual identity in preservation of self with Alzheimer's. *Journal of Religion, Spirituality, and Aging, 26,* 65–91.

37 McFadden, J. T. (2012). *Aging, dementia, and the faith community: Continuing the journey of friendship.* Eugene, OR: Wipf & Stock. Accessed on 9/15/19 at http://d1swb5ay1qopx0.cloudfront.net/wp-content/uploads/2016/07/EP-pamphlet-16.pdf

38 Goldsmith, M. (2004, July/August). Spirituality, religion and faith in dementia care. *Journal of Dementia Care, 12*(4), 28–30. (p. 29)

39 Kimble, M. A., McFadden, S. H., Ellor, J. W., & Seeber, J. J. (Eds.). (1995). *Aging, religion, and spirituality: A handbook.* Minneapolis, MN: Fortress Press.

40 Kimble, M. A., & McFadden, S. H. (Eds.). (2002). *Aging, religion, and spirituality: A handbook* (Vol. 2). Minneapolis, MN: Fortress Press.

41 Everett, D. (1999). Forget me not: The spiritual care of people with Alzheimer's disease. *Journal of Health Care Chaplaincy, 8*(1/2), 77–88.

42 Everett, p. 87.

43 www.bls.gov/ooh/healthcare/nursing-assistants.htm

44 https://aspe.hhs.gov/2019-poverty-guidelines

45 Goldsmith, M. (2004). *In a strange land: People with dementia and the local church.* Edinburgh, UK: 4M Publications. (p. 172)

Part 5

EMBRACING THE NEW STORY

Chapter 11

Sustaining Dignity, Hope, and Meaning in the Time of Dementia

Everyone has a complex, multi-faceted life story with themes of joy and sorrow, love gained and love lost, success and disappointment, health and illness. But it seems that for many people, once the dementia diagnosis enters the story, the lighter parts fade and only darkness remains. At least, that is how it is often interpreted by other people, even though persons with the diagnosis may continue to experience multiple sources of meaning, be blessed by having their dignity affirmed by others, and retain the ability to hold on to hope. The tragedy narrative may swirl around them and those who love them, but it can recede to the background because of a new story being told worldwide—a story about community inclusion and support, human rights, and support for sustaining psychological and social well-being throughout the dementia journey.

Yes, the big numbers about dementia are frightening. To cite just one more example, in Japan—which is sometimes described as a super-aged society—by 2025 there will be over seven million people living with a dementia.[1] That represents about 5.5 percent of the total population (compared with the United States where about 1.8 percent of the population currently lives with a dementia[2]). That country has adopted national and local dementia-friendly and inclusive community initiatives involving government, non-governmental organizations, and local groups. They have developed well-organized, effective programs to educate citizens about the dementias, eliminate the stigma, ensure inclusion of people living with the condition in decision-making, and creatively develop programs and services supporting the best possible life quality.[3] Of course, Japan is a country with a long and rich tradition of honoring not only their elders but also community life as a whole.

Other countries that have woven their national stories around rugged individualism—the US being the largest and most obvious example—are just now realizing the need to develop stronger community ties to help people resist the physical and mental health challenges that come with the loneliness, boredom, and helplessness prevalent in aging people, especially those living with a dementia. This individualism can have harmful effects on diagnosed persons who refuse to acknowledge that they have become more vulnerable and dependent on others. It can also be harmful to care partners who will not ask for help from their families, their friends and neighbors, their community organizations, or their governments. Although we like to deny this, as human beings we are all vulnerable; we need to seek interdependence rather than independence and rely on others for much of what makes our life good. And yet too many people abide by an old saying my mother often repeated: "You should not air your dirty linen." Sadly, this belief prevented her from getting any help for the care she gave my father for over 10 years, until finally, at the end of his life, he had to be moved to a nursing home.

Even in the US, with its national pride in innovation, independence, and individual achievement, there is widespread and honest acknowledgment that for baby boomers and their parents, there will probably be no medical intervention that can cure the various types of dementia. For the next 30 years, when nations around the world will be contending with high numbers of frail elders, a different approach to dementia will be necessary, one that replaces the fantasy of medical science coming to the rescue. Of course, we may see a remarkable breakthrough in developing easily identifiable biomarkers present in young and middle-aged adults that reliably predict future development of some type of dementia. Ideally, this identification would be inexpensive, noninvasive, and available to everyone, with some kind of guaranteed treatment to follow that would also be inexpensive, noninvasive, and available to everyone. Perhaps there will be affordable vaccines for each type of dementia so that everyone born in the second half of the twenty-first century will never have to worry about developing dementia symptoms. However, between now and that fantasized future, what can we do? A new story will have to energize the imaginations of government leaders and citizens, a new story not propelled by dread (which increases the stigma afflicting people with the diagnosis) but rather by faith in the good will of people who want their communities to be places that nourish a meaningful life for everyone.

People all over the world are beginning to tell this new story. Many have some type of diagnosed dementia or love someone with the diagnosis. They are stepping up as advocates and activists, not content to go along with the expectation that they should disappear from community life. They are disrupting the idea that once you get a diagnosis (which is now coming earlier, especially for wealthier people who have decent health insurance and can pay for tests not covered by Medicare) you should just step off life's stage, get out of the way, and fade away. They are disrupting the failure to acknowledge the human rights of people living with dementia, regardless of where they happen to be on the spectrum of dementia progression. They are disrupting the assumption that the millions—billions—of dollars needed for biomedical research will cure all types of dementia. Some may even disrupt the prejudice that all long-term-care communities are horrible, smelly, depressing places where no one would want a loved one to live (though, of course, some are still that way, and the disruption will come when people challenge the poor care that too often is the only option for poor people).

All of these disruptions may remind people that the times are "a-changing." We no longer talk about senility, and we are beginning to understand that there are many types of dementia besides Alzheimer's disease. More organizations that operate long-term care residences are accepting new culture practices that affirm and support the personhood of residents as well as staff (who are still woefully underpaid and lack important training in caring for people with dementia). Although there is a worldwide push for dementia to be viewed as a disability, and although there has been progress in the US in obtaining disability benefits for people diagnosed in midlife, some still resist putting people with dementia in the same category as those born with intellectual or developmental disabilities, or as people whose sensory or motor disability comes at birth or later in life. Nevertheless, a commitment to protecting the human rights of people living with dementia is growing, as seen in documents produced by national governments, international and national non-profit organizations, and groups operating on a regional level.

Much of the work to raise awareness of the need for a new story about dementia has come from individuals living with dementia joining forces in organizations such as Dementia Friendly America, Alzheimer Europe, and Alzheimer's Disease International (which consists of dementia advocacy organizations from 95 countries). These and other organizations like them model dementia inclusiveness. They are committed to having people living with dementia join their boards, chair symposia at their conferences, participate in videos on their websites, and in many other ways make their voices heard.

Many people who spoke up and out about various political and cultural issues when they were teens and young adults will undoubtedly continue to do that as they age into elderhood. They have already seen some of their musical icons, such as Glen Campbell, reveal a dementia diagnosis; in the coming years, more well-known cultural figures are likely to follow the role models mentioned in Chapter 4 and go public with their diagnoses. Some people will wear T-shirts proclaiming things like "I have Alzheimer's. Deal with it!" They want their communities to offer opportunities to continue to be employed or to volunteer to serve others in some way. After all, we now have decades of research showing that voluntarism is good for people's mental and physical health, especially after retirement. People living with a dementia want to be able to continue to engage in ordinary interactions in their communities, such as grocery shopping, using public transportation, going to the library, and eating in restaurants.

People with a dementia diagnosis also want their health-care systems to be dementia capable with compassionate, patient providers and easy-to-negotiate physical environments. In the US, despite all the arguing by politicians about how to pay for health care, one never hears an older person say "give me all the resources; leave none for children." Indeed, if more resources went into public-health efforts across the lifespan to encourage healthier eating, more exercise, greater social engagement, better education, more cognitive stimulation, and other empirically validated ways of improving brain health, it would represent a boon not just for older people but also for the health of everyone, regardless of age. Other examples come from public-health efforts to reduce traumatic brain injuries. These include encouraging people to wear helmets, addressing potential for domestic violence before it occurs, changing rules in sports with high risk of head injuries, and eliminating homelessness (which raises the risk of head injuries, or may be caused by head injuries). Again, these efforts help people of all ages be healthier citizens and may even, in some cases, reduce the prevalence of certain types of dementia.

Along with public-health campaigns, the worldwide effort to train people to be Dementia Friends is spreading, with some countries, such as Japan, actively encouraging Dementia Friends to support people with dementia to remain included in social events in their villages, towns, and cities. Intergenerational programs are becoming more popular as people witness the joy of elders and young people spending time together, often doing something creative. Community education programs are helping people retain friendship connections even when a friend begins to forget details about the friendship. And a few people are beginning to address the reasons behind the breakdown of relationships that lead to social rejection and even bullying. They are attempting to ameliorate these painful encounters through educational programs that increase knowledge about the ways in which dementia affects emotions and behaviors.

Just as people living with dementia, their family members, and friends are reimagining how villages, towns, and cities can be more hospitable to people with dementia symptoms, some are also reimagining new models of residential care communities. Recognizing that these may be the best option for an individual who can no longer live safely and well in a private home environment, some organizations are creating living spaces that encourage and support expressions of agency. For example, people who live in these new models of residential care are encouraged to wake up and eat breakfast when they want to; choose a bath over a shower, if that is what they prefer; skip bingo, if they don't enjoy it; and sit outside on a beautiful day, if that is what draws them. These memory-care communities have staff trained to discern what people are attempting to communicate through behaviors such as shouting, crying, and hitting. Their administrators get to know the residents and encourage the development of social connections among residents and residents' families and friends. In other words, they are community builders.

This kind of care is expensive, available in some countries to wealthy people, as well as to less affluent people fortunate enough to have some savings. In the US, whether a person with dementia lives in a long-term-care community or in a private home or apartment, the costs of care in the last five years of life far exceed the costs of caring for someone with cancer or heart disease. One study found that out-of-pocket spending (that is, expenses not covered by Medicare and supplemental insurance) for someone with dementia is on average 81 percent higher than for people the same age who do not live with dementia. Although some home health-care expenses in the US may be covered by Medicare—in particular, services such as physical and occupational therapy for recovery from an acute health crisis—families receive little or no outside financial support to hire a home-care aide to assist with tasks such as meal preparation and house cleaning.[4] And only about 10 percent of Americans over age 62 have private long-term-care insurance,[5] which can normally be activated once a person needs assistance with two or more "activities of daily living" (which include tasks such as eating, dressing, and bathing but exclude tasks such as shopping, cooking, and cleaning) or if the person needs supervision for their safety, which may be most relevant for a person in the middle stage of dementia.

The question of payment for medical care, along with social care such as adult day services and practical in-home care that might delay the need to relocate to some type of long-term-care community, must be addressed by government leaders willing to accept that current policies and payment systems will be insufficient to meet the needs of aging persons in the next 30 years. Discussion of how to pay for all the modifications required for communities truly to be dementia aware, capable, enabling, friendly, inclusive, positive, and supportive can quickly devolve into political fights over distribution of resources to cover all of the pressing issues we face today. Too many people see this as a zero-sum game; they believe, for example, that we can only have

- good schools (including preschools) for all children *or* good care for their grandparents and great-grandparents

- more roads for personal vehicles (that many older people can no longer use) *or* improved public transportation

- affordable health care for all *or* lower taxes.

Resolving these conflicts will require political leadership from people willing to work together regardless of party affiliation in order to define priorities and how to pay for them. Tragically, that kind of leadership worldwide appears to be in short supply today.

Another way of stating this is that creating communities for people to live well with dementia is not only a matter of good-hearted people being trained as Dementia Friends, starting memory cafés, offering regular educational programs, surveying their cities and towns to determine whether they can be safely navigated, or enlisting businesses in learning how to communicate helpfully with people living with dementia. All these actions, and more, are important for community groups that come together for the purpose of funding, planning, and enacting these dementia-friendly and inclusive community initiatives. However, citizens also need to advocate for public policy at the local, regional, and national level in order to address the structural fracture points that impose so much burden on families and persons with dementia.

Discussions about the many medical, financial, and social challenges of life with dementia can quickly take one down a path with no illumination of moments of joy and playfulness. This is one reason why it is important to continually remind people of the role of the arts in dementia-friendly and inclusive communities. Although painters, poets, writers, musicians, and other artists often creatively invite people to gaze into the shadows of human lives, they can also pour beauty, awe, and wonder into life. Engagement with art forms of all kinds not only supports the goal of a good life for those touched by dementia but also offers a different vision of life with dementia for people in the wider community whose only image focuses on deterioration and loss.

As Anne Basting has written, "The experience of memory loss is gray. We need to get comfortable in the gray and keep our eyes and hearts open for moments of grace."[6]

Living with dementia, whether as a diagnosed person, a care partner, family member, or friend, necessitates maneuvering through this gray zone, a place where the joys of human life mix with its sorrows. The task is hard, and the people willing to accept life in the gray zone are tremendously courageous. Their defiant human spirit will not be extinguished by the hardships imposed on them by the brain changes of dementia.

Similarly, Basting's moments of grace are what Janet Ramsey had in mind when she wrote about "tough hope." Tough hope "acknowledges the terrifying landscape of dementia and the daily challenges of tests, doctors' visits, medications, and constant decline." But tough hope also offers "glimpses of a different kind of dream"[7] in which there are redemptive moments in the present and, for followers of certain religious faiths, assurance of the enduring and abiding love of God.

Someday, even without cures for all the types of dementia, the practices and policies of dementia-friendliness and dementia-inclusivity may be intimately woven into the whole life of our communities. The ideal would be to embrace ways of living together in community that are friendly toward and inclusive of *all* persons. Making communities good for people living with dementia can make them good for everyone.

Endnotes

1   McCurry, J. (2018, January 15). "Dementia towns": How Japan is evolving for its ageing population. *The Guardian.* Accessed on 4/14/20 at www.theguardian.com/world/2018/jan/15/dementia-towns-japan-ageing-population

2   This percentage was obtained by dividing the Alzheimer's Association's frequently cited figure of 5.5 million people living with dementia in the US by the total population in the US.

3   For a description of how one city in Japan began a dementia-friendly city initiative in 1990, see https://www.alz.co.uk/dementia-friendly-communities/uji

4   Kelley, A. S., McGarry, K., Gorges, R., & Skinner, J. S. (2015). The burden of health care costs for patients with dementia in the last five years of life. *Annals of Internal Medicine, 163,* 729–736.

5   Braun, R. A., Kopecky, K. A., & Koreshkova, T. (2019). Old, frail, and uninsured: Accounting for features of the U.S. long-term care insurance market. *Econometrica, 87,* 981–1019.

6   Basting, A. D. (2009). *Forget memory: Creating better lives for people with dementia.* Baltimore, MD: Johns Hopkins University Press. (p. 156)

7   Ramsey, J. (2018). *Dignity and grace: Wisdom for caregivers and those living with dementia.* Minneapolis, MN: Fortress Press. (p. 152)

Dementia-Friendly and Inclusive Communities and Memory Cafés

General Information
Alzheimer's Society (UK)

www.alzheimers.org.uk/categories/campaigns/dementia-friendly-communities

This page gives links to many documents about dementia-friendly communities. The one called "Building Dementia-Friendly Communities: A Priority for Everyone" is based on interviews with people with dementia about what they most wanted from their communities.

Checklists for Developing Dementia-Friendly Communities

www.housinglin.org.uk/_library/Resources/Housing/Support_materials/Viewpoints/Viewpoint25_AtAGlance.pdf

This document deals primarily with environmental design that can help make communities more welcoming and easier to navigate for people with memory loss and confusion.

Dementia Action Alliance

https://daanow.org

The DAA supports people living with dementia and care partners in advocacy efforts to create dementia-friendly communities.

Dementia Friendly America

www.dfamerica.org

This national organization grew out of the Minnesota Act on Alzheimer's work. It sponsors the Dementia Friends program that is spreading through the US. In 2017, Minnesota trained 10,000 people to be Dementia Friends.

Minnesota ACT on Alzheimer's

www.actonalz.org

This organization developed a detailed toolkit to help communities assess how dementia capable they are. It includes information about memory cafés.

Wisconsin Healthy Brain Initiative

www.dhs.wisconsin.gov/publications/p01000.pdf

The Wisconsin Department of Health Services developed this dementia-friendly community toolkit.

Regional Dementia-Friendly Communities
Dementia-Inclusive Durham

www.facebook.com/dementiainclusivedurham

This new organization in Durham, NC, does not have a website at this time, but its Facebook page gives a lot of information about its local efforts to form and fund collaborations to create dementia inclusion in the region.

Fox Valley Memory Project

www.foxvalleymemoryproject.org

A regional effort in northeast Wisconsin, Fox Valley Memory Project serves people living with dementia and their care partners from the time they first worry about their memory and other cognitive functions through the progression of their condition. It is best known for its memory cafés but it has many other programs that provide opportunities for social connectedness.

Momentia

www.momentiaseattle.org

Momentia is a grassroots effort to create dementia-friendly and inclusive communities in the Puget Sound region of Washington State. The website contains testimonies from people living with dementia and descriptions of regional events featuring a range of activities from singing to zoo visits and garden walks.

Information about Memory Cafés
The Alzheimer's Café

www.thirdageservices.com/AlzCafe%20handbook.pdf

This PDF has much practical information about starting and operating cafés and includes comments from a survey of 11 memory cafés around the country about what worked well and some problems encountered in operating memory cafés.

Alzheimer's Cafés and Memory Cafés

www.alzheimerscafe.com/public.html.alzheimersatoz.com/ Welcome.html

This site compares the evolving models of Alzheimer's cafés and memory cafés and contains many practical suggestions for starting and running memory cafés.

Massachusetts Memory Café Toolkit

www.jfcsboston.org/MemoryCafeToolkit

Jewish Family & Children's Service, an organization that now coordinates over 100 memory cafés throughout Massachusetts, developed this guide. It is notable for including information about inclusive and specialized cafés serving people with hearing loss, younger-onset dementia, and intellectual/developmental disorders. It also describes cafés for LGBTQ persons and offers advice for developing culture/language-specific cafés.

This toolkit has been translated into Spanish: www.jfcsboston.org/GuiaCafeDeMemoria

Memory Café Catalyst

http://memorycafecatalyst.org

This is an online community offering information and support for persons involved with memory cafés; some are just beginning cafés and some have been operating them for several years. The site includes a document in Spanish about memory cafés that were developed in Lawrence, MA.

Memory Café Directory

www.memorycafedirectory.com

This interactive page gives information about memory cafés in each state in the US.

Neighborhood Memory Café Tool Kit

www.thirdageservices.com/Memory%20Cafe%20Tool%20Kit.pdf

This brief document published in 2012 contains practical advice for starting and sustaining a memory café.

Rotarians Easing Problems of Dementia

www.repod.org.uk

Rotary Clubs in England provided early leadership and support for memory cafés. They published the original guide for setting up a memory café and continue to use their website to promote memory cafés and ideas for creating dementia-friendly communities.

Wisconsin Memory Cafés: A Best Practice Guide

https://wai.wisc.edu/best-practice-guides

Like several other toolkits describing how to create and sustain memory cafés, this document offers helpful information for local groups seeking to establish one or more memory cafés.

Acknowledgments

In all the chapters of this book, I have shared ideas gleaned from journal articles, books, newspaper articles, and websites. Close friends published some of them, but most came from people I will never meet. All have been my teachers. They have contributed to my understanding of how we might create dementia-friendly and inclusive communities and why we need to do this. Now it is my privilege to acknowledge some of my other teachers.

I must start with people living with dementia, beginning with memory-care residents of the Evergreen retirement community in Oshkosh, Wisconsin, where I first experienced the joys of facilitating TimeSlips creative-storytelling sessions almost 20 years ago. Equally important to my education over the years are all the people who generously invited my students and me into their homes so we could conduct interviews and ask them to complete various scales and questionnaires. I also cherish as friends and teachers the participants in Fox Valley Memory Project memory cafés and its chorus. They have taught me just as much about living as well as possible with dementia as all those books and journal articles I have hauled back and forth between my home in Appleton, Wisconsin, and my cabin in the Upper Peninsula of Michigan.

I am grateful for friends around the world who have championed dementia-friendly and inclusive communities: in England, Linda Clare, Rob Merchant, and Jane Moore; in Switzerland and Canada, Rebecca Giselbrecht; in Australia, Elizabeth MacKinlay; in Germany, Karin Wilkening; and in Poland, Dr. Katarzyna Broczek. Likewise, I have been inspired by many people in the US, including Marigrace Becker, Dr. Abhilash Desai, Emily Farah-Miller, Dayle Friedman,

Maria Genné, Gary Glazner, Lori LaBey, Jytte Lokvig, Karen Love, Keri Pollock, Janet Ramsey, Marty Richards, and Beth Soltzberg.

Had I not been asked by the dean of my college in 1996 to be a mentor to a new faculty member in the English department, my life would have taken a very different turn. That was the year I met Anne Basting. I count her as one of my closest friends and most significant teachers.

I feel fortunate to live in Wisconsin, a source of considerable national leadership and inspiration for the formation of dementia-friendly and inclusive communities. The SPARK Alliance of arts and cultural institutions serving people living with dementia has been a particular source of joy and learning for me. Bader Philanthropies in Milwaukee supported the establishment of the SPARK Alliance as well as Fox Valley Memory Project and many of the creative programs designed by Anne Basting. People working in the Wisconsin Department of Health Services and at the Wisconsin Alzheimer's Institute have also played an important role in promoting progressive approaches to creating friendly, inclusive communities for people living with dementia.

I have lived in Appleton since 1983 and have had the good fortune of forming friendships with many people in our beautiful corner of the world. Anca, Andrea, Anna, Barb, Barry, Beth, Bob, Bonnie, Brad, Cristinel, Ellie, Esther, Franny, Jeff, Jim, Jonathan, Jone, Nancy, Sandra, Sean, and Tom have been especially close and supportive of my work.

Since 1985, I have had the privilege of working with students at the University of Wisconsin–Oshkosh who took my classes on aging and signed up for independent study, service learning, and research assistantships in order to learn more about how to enhance the lives of people living with dementia. Three who were especially helpful as I organized materials for this book were Heather Flick, Alexandra Ebert, and Amy Hodel.

In addition, this book would have been very different without the assistance of Martha Stettinius of MS Edits. She not only had me thinking about gerunds for the first time since high school but also offered many useful suggestions to help me keep my readers engaged. Having written her own book about caring for her mother who lived with dementia, Martha offered important insights as well into current issues in dementia research, practice, and policy.

Finally, I must acknowledge my husband, John, who drove those 860 miles in England so we could experience memory cafés firsthand and then joined me in establishing them in our part of Wisconsin. He has been actively involved with Fox Valley Memory Project since its inception and spreads joy in local nursing homes where he plays his ukulele and engages residents in singing familiar songs. He has helped me carry multiple bags of books and files back and forth between our home and our cabin, and he has gently reminded me to stand up, move around, and drink water when I became too fixated on my writing. For all this and so much more, I thank him.

Index